THE FACTS ABOUT ALTERNATIVE MEDICINE

TIME LIFE
BOOKS

Time-Life Books - UK
Publisher: Helen Wicks
Managing Editor: Mark Stephenson
Editor: Nancy Duin
Editorial: Kate Cann

Time-Life Books - US
Director of Editorial Development: Jennifer Pearce
Editor: Robert Somerville
Deputy Editor: Tina S. McDowell
Design Director: Tina Taylor
Text Editor: Jim Watson
Associate Editors/Research and Writing: Nancy Blodgett, Stephanie
Summers Henke
Technical Art Assistant: Dana R. Magsumbol
Senior Copyeditors: Anne Farr, Mary Beth Oelkers-Keegan
Picture Coordinator: Lisa Groseclose
Editorial Assistant: Patricia D. Whiteford

ISBN 0-7054-3025-1

The textual and visual decriptions of medical conditions and treatment options in this book should be considered as a reference source only; they are not intended to substitute for a medical diagnosis, advice, and treatment. Always consult your doctor or other qualified practitioner for proper medical care.

Before using any drug or natural medicine mentioned in this book, be sure to check with your doctor, and examine carefully the product packaging or other reliable source of information for any warnings or cautions. You should keep in mind that herbal remedies are not as strictly regulated as drugs.

Cover photographs courtesy of PhotoDisc
Cover design by Anna Burgard

Table of Contents

Introduction

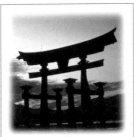

Good health is more than an absence of illness. Alternative medicine understands how the body, mind and spirit work together to help you feel well, and heal. This book offers explanations and safety information for a wide variety of alternative treatments to let you know what your options are in addition to the traditional drugs and surgeries of conventional medicine.

In the following pages, 29 forms of therapy are arranged by name in alphabetical order. Most are listed individually, but in some cases a few similar or related techniques are grouped under a single umbrella heading. Body work, for instance, is a general category for therapies that involve bodily manipulation or techniques for improving posture and movement. (Note: Massage and chiropractic, though generally considered to be body work techniques, are listed separately.) Therapies that rely on the healing power of the mind—biofeedback, guided imagery, and hypnotherapy, to name a few—are discussed under the group heading Mind/Body Medicine. If you're not sure where to look for a particular therapy, you can find it easily in the index.

Each entry offers a comprehensive, 'big picture' look at a given therapy as well as a close examination of its various elements. An introduction sets the stage, defining the technique and explaining its working principles. Next comes a brief review of the technique's historical origins, identifying the key players and explaining how their methods evolved over the decades or millennia into the therapy as practised today.

Under 'What It's Good For', you'll find general information about how this therapy acts on the body to improve health. Specific disorders commonly treated with this method are listed as 'Target Ailments'. 'Preparations/Techniques' delves into the nuts and bolts of the therapy; here you'll learn such things as how healing substances are prepared and administered, and what techniques or equipment is used. Under 'Visiting a Professional', you'll find out what you can expect when visiting a practitioner's office. Because well-being is a big part of alternative medicine, most entries describe how a given therapy helps promote and maintain lasting good health. 'What the Critics Say' attempts to characterize—and occasionally rebut—criticisms that have been levelled against this form of therapy. A box labelled 'For More Info' lists the contact details of organizations you can get in touch with to learn more about the topic.

Also featured are illustrated galleries that give practical, in-depth information about selected remedies and therapeutic techniques. The acupressure gallery, for example, shows exactly how and where to apply healing pressure to the body for relaxation and good health. Another gallery provides step-by-step instruction in therapeutic massage, while others explore such health-related topics as vitamins and minerals, herbs, essential oils and homoeopathic remedies.

How to Choose a Practitioner

When searching for an alternative practitioner, you may want to begin with a recommendation from a conventional doctor. Illness-related self-help groups and books on alternative healing can also be good sources for names. You may find that family and friends can provide valuable opinions based on their experience with particular practitioners. In your search, don't hesitate to act on personal considerations such as a preference for a male or female practitioner, or an older or younger one. If you have beliefs or philosophies that play a major role in your healthcare, be sure that you choose a provider who will respect your views.

You should fully investigate any alternative practitioner's background and experience and check if he or she is registered with any professional organization and whether he or she has insurance. Be extremely suspicious of anyone who expresses hostility or derision toward mainstream medicine or makes grandiose claims for a cure. A conscientious practitioner understands that every therapy has its limitations. Get explicit information about the treatment you will receive, and remember that you are in charge of the entire treatment process. Above all, trust your own instincts and judgment. ■

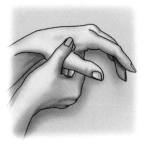

Target Ailments

- Allergies
- Arthritis
- Asthma
- Athletic Injuries
- Back Problems
- Chronic Fatigue Syndrome
- Common Cold
- Constipation
- Diarrhoea
- Earache
- Headache
- Immune Problems
- Indigestion
- Insomnia
- Motion Sickness
- Nausea
- Pain, Chronic
- TMJ Syndrome
- Toothache

Acupressure

A *n integral part of the traditional practice of Chinese medicine (pages 45-48), acupressure has become increasingly popular and accepted in the West. Its simple, non-invasive techniques have shown beneficial effects for a wide array of health problems—even if the theory behind it remains questionable to many conventional medical practitioners.*

Like acupuncture (pages 22-23), acupressure is based on the concept of chi (sometimes spelled 'qi'), defined in Chinese medicine as an essential life force that flows through the body, circulating through invisible passageways called meridians (see the illustrations on pages 24-25). The movement, or flow, of chi is said to vary with the mental, physical and spiritual changes of daily living. According to this theory, when chi flows freely and evenly, harmony and good health are possible; however, if chi circulation is stagnant, overstimulated or unbalanced, illness is likely.

The invisible meridians carrying chi are said to reside within the body's interior. However, there are specific places on the skin, called acupoints, where chi may be accessed and guided using deep, focused finger pressure. By improving chi circulation, practitioners encourage the harmonious equilibrium of mind and body believed to be essential for physical and spiritual health. And once this internal harmony is achieved, they claim, the body is able to invoke its self-healing capabilities.

Origins

The various therapeutic techniques of Chinese medicine, including acupressure, are among the most ancient healing approaches in the world, dating back some 5,000 years. Acupressure itself probably originated as a combination of acupuncture and massage.

What It's Good For

Acupressure techniques address hundreds of ailments. In addition to those listed at left, studies have shown that acupressure can hasten recuperation from stroke and surgery. And at some hospitals, elastic acupressure wristbands (designed to relieve motion sickness) are used to reduce the anaesthesia-induced nausea that often follows surgery. Acupressure can also be valuable during pregnancy, as it may relieve morning sickness, indigestion and backache; alleviate the pain of childbirth; and enhance recuperation. But be sure to read the caution at right.

Acupressure

Preparations/Techniques

Acupressure can be performed by a trained specialist or by patients in their own homes. A specialist can provide comprehensive treatment, which involves the redirecting of chi around the meridians; the British Acupuncture Council can help you locate a good practitioner. To try acupressure yourself for local, symptomatic relief, you will first need to identify which acupoints are best suited for your specific ailment, preferably with the help of an acupressure practitioner. This may be a single point, or several points in a specific order. Locate the first acupoint *(using the Gallery of Acupressure Techniques, pages 8-21)* and press lightly with one finger. Gradually increase the pressure until you are comfortably pressing as firmly as you can. Hold this pressure steadily until you begin to feel a very faint, even pulse at the acupoint. (This usually takes three to 10 minutes, or longer for severe problems.) When you're ready to release, reduce the pressure from the acupoint very slowly. You may occasionally feel some discomfort, but if the pressure is actually painful, ease up. There is no 'correct' amount of pressure that you should strive for; everyone's needs are different, and the amount required at one acupoint will vary from that needed at another.

For best results, apply pressure to the same acupoints on both sides of the body; when working with a series of acupoints, complete the set on one side of the body before continuing to the other side. In some forms of acupressure, such as shiatsu, pressure is applied sequentially, from one end of the meridian to the other. To work on hard-to-reach spots (such as your back), either ask a partner for help, or place a tennis or golf ball on the floor and then lie on top of it.

Well-being

Beyond its many potential healing effects, acupressure may also be beneficial in maintaining overall good health. Acupressure releases tension in muscle fibres, promoting the movement of blood and nutrients to the tissues. Many people report acupressure induces peaceful rejuvenation and clarity of thought, as well as improved athletic performance.

What the Critics Say

Because no one is certain just how acupressure works, its critics typically claim that it is simply not effective, offering the placebo effect to explain its success. Studies testing the placebo effect do not support this criticism, however. ■

CAUTION

If you have a serious illness, ask your doctor before using acupressure. Never press on an open wound, swollen or inflamed skin, bruises, varicose veins or a lump. Avoid sites of recent surgery and sites of a suspected bone injury. If you have atherosclerosis, avoid direct pressure on the carotid arteries. If you are pregnant, avoid pressure to the lower abdomen, and don't use points Spleen 6 or Large Intestine 4 (some believe these points can induce miscarriage).

FOR MORE INFO
Following is a list of organizations you can contact to learn more about acupressure:

British Acupuncture Council
63 Jeddo Road
London W12 9HQ
020 8735 0400
fax: 020 8735 0404

Institute for Complementary Medicine
PO Box 194
London SE16 1QZ
fax: 020 7237 5175

Gallery of Acupressure Techniques

Bladder 10

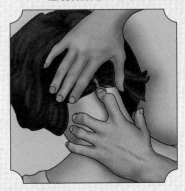

■ Locate the ropy muscles 0.5 in (1 cm) below the base of the skull. Press inwards using the thumb or a finger.

Bladder 13

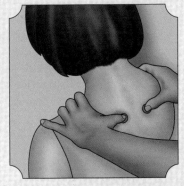

■ Use your thumbs or fingers to press into the muscles 0.5 in (1 cm) outwards from either side of the spine and one finger width below the upper tip of the shoulder blade.

Bladder 23

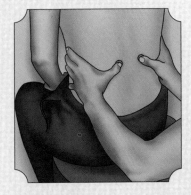

■ This point site is level with the space between the second and third lumbar vertebrae. Find BL 23 by aligning your thumbs or fingers about 1 in (2.5 cm) outwards from either side of the spine, just behind the navel, then press inwards.

Bladder 25

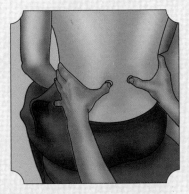

■ With your thumbs or fingers, press into the muscles about 1 in (2.5 cm) outward from either side of the spine, about midway between BL 23 (left) and the bottom of the spine. The point is level with the fourth and fifth lumbar vertebrae.

Gallery of Acupressure Techniques

Bladder 32

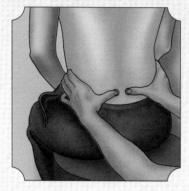

■ At the base of the spine, directly above the tail-bone, use your thumbs or fingers to press into the muscles 0.5 in (1 cm) outwards from either side of the spine.

Bladder 40

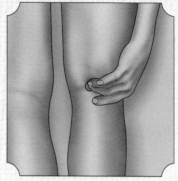

■ With your leg slightly bent, find the fold on the back of your knee where the knee bends. Use your middle finger to press inwards on the fold, between the two tendons.

Conception Vessel 4

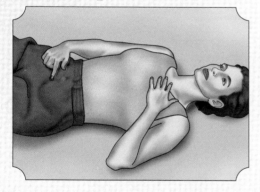

■ Locate this point, which lies just below CV 6 (right), by measuring four finger widths down from the navel on the midline of the abdomen. With your index finger, gradually press as deep as possible on the point site.

Conception Vessel 6

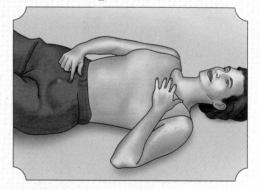

■ Measure three finger widths below the navel—or about one finger width up from CV 4 (left)—then press inwards on this point as far as you can, using your index finger. Inhale slowly and deeply, relaxing as you exhale.

CONTINUED

Gallery of Acupressure Techniques

Conception Vessel 12

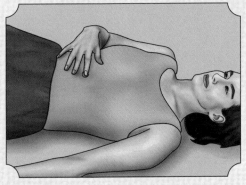

■ This point lies four thumb widths above the navel along the midline of the belly, about halfway between the navel and the bottom of the breastbone. Press softly inwards, using your index finger.

Conception Vessel 17

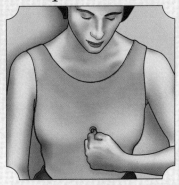

■ Place your index finger in the centre of your chest, midway between the nipples, and press lightly.

Conception Vessel 22

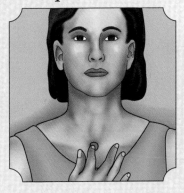

■ This point lies directly below the Adam's apple, midway between the collarbones in the large hollow at the base of the throat. Place the tip of your index or middle finger on the point site and press downwards lightly.

Gall Bladder 2

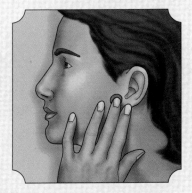

■ Open your mouth and, feeling along the jawbone, locate the depression directly in front of your ears. Place the tips of your middle fingers about 0.5 in (1 cm) below the base of the depression. Close your mouth and press steadily on the point.

Gallery of Acupressure Techniques

Gall Bladder 20

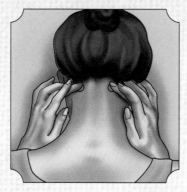

■ Place the tips of your middle fingers in the hollows at the base of your skull, about 2 in (5 cm) apart on either side of the spine. Press firmly.

Gall Bladder 21

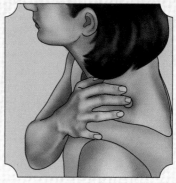

■ Apply pressure with your right middle finger to the highest point on your left shoulder muscle, 1–2 in (2.5–5 cm) out from the base of the neck. Repeat on the other side. (Use light pressure if you are pregnant.)

Gall Bladder 34

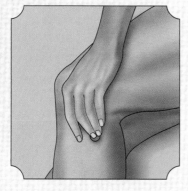

■ While seated with legs bent, locate the bony indentation on your lower leg just below and to the outside of the kneecap. Apply firm pressure to the point with your finger or thumb.

Gall Bladder 39

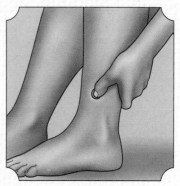

■ To find this point, measure four finger widths above the outside anklebone, in front of the fibula, on the lower leg. Apply pressure with the tip of your finger or thumb.

CONTINUED

Gallery of Acupressure Techniques

Governing Vessel 4

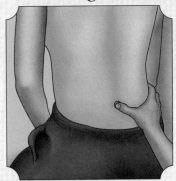

■ Press hard with your thumb on the midline of the spine, directly behind the navel. The point is located between the second and third lumbar vertebrae.

Governing Vessel 14

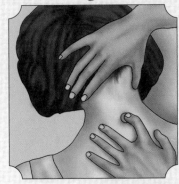

■ Tilt your head and locate the seventh cervical vertebra, the most prominent bone on the back of your neck. Have a helper press the thumb or index finger hard between this bone and the first thoracic vertebra below it.

Governing Vessel 20

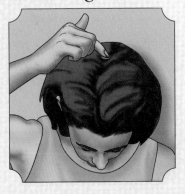

■ This point is located on the flat spot at the top of the head, midway along an imaginary line connecting the upper part of the ears. Apply pressure with your thumb or index finger. (Do not press this point if you have high blood pressure.)

Governing Vessel 24.5

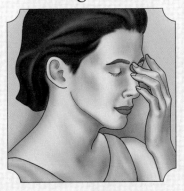

■ Place the tip of your middle finger at the top of the bridge of the nose, between your eyebrows. Press lightly.

Gallery of Acupressure Techniques

Governing Vessel 25

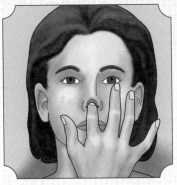

▇ Lightly press the tip of your nose with the end of your finger.

Heart 3

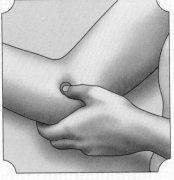

▇ On the inside of the upper arm, use your thumb to apply pressure next to the tendon in the indentation near the inside elbow crease, in line with the little finger.

Heart 7

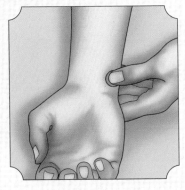

▇ This point is located on the crease along the inside of the wrist, directly in line with the little finger. Squeeze firmly, using the thumb and index finger of your other hand.

Kidney 1

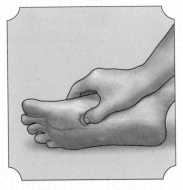

▇ Use one or both thumbs to press just behind the ball of the foot, in the slight indentation of the back of the large pad that corresponds to the big toe. (Do not use this point if you have low blood pressure.)

CONTINUED

Gallery of Acupressure Techniques

Kidney 3

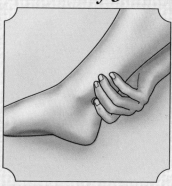

▪ This point lies midway between the inside anklebone and the Achilles tendon at the back of
the ankle. Apply pressure with your thumb or
index finger. (Avoid using this point after the third
month of pregnancy.)

Large Intestine 4

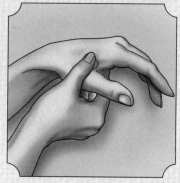

▪ Use the thumb and index finger of your right
hand to squeeze the webbing between the thumb
and index finger of your left hand. Switch hands
and repeat. (Do not apply pressure to this point if
you are pregnant.)

Large Intestine 10

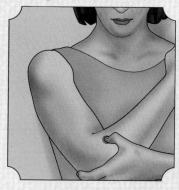

▪ With your arm bent and your palm down, measure two thumb widths below the edge of the elbow
crease. The point site lies in the groove between
the muscles on the outside of the arm. Press hard
with your thumb, then repeat on the other arm.

Large Intestine 11

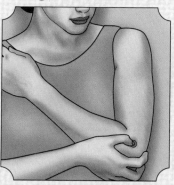

▪ With your arm bent, use your thumb to press
deeply on the outer edge of the elbow crease.
Repeat on the other arm.

Gallery of Acupressure Techniques

Large Intestine 20

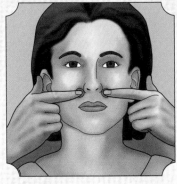

■ Using your index or middle fingers, press hard on the outer edge of the nostrils at the base of the nose.

Liver 2

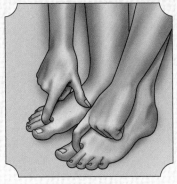

■ On the top of each foot, use your index finger to press into the webbing between the big toe and the second toe.

Liver 3

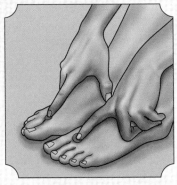

■ Place your index fingers next to the large knuckle of each big toe, then press into the groove on top of the foot between the big toe and the second toe.

Liver 8

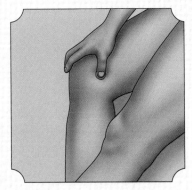

■ Bend the right knee and place your right thumb just above the knee crease on the inside of the leg. The point lies just below the knee joint (swing your leg a few times to help locate it). Press, then repeat on the other leg.

CONTINUED

Gallery of Acupressure Techniques

Lung 1

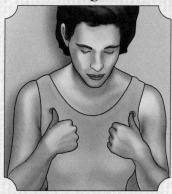

■ Place the thumb or index finger of each hand about 0.5 in (1 cm) below the large hollow under the collarbone, on the outer part of the chest near the shoulder. Apply pressure gently.

Lung 5

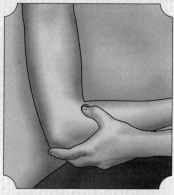

■ Bend your right elbow and make a fist. Place your left thumb on the outside crease (thumb side) of the elbow alongside the taut tendon and press firmly. Repeat on the other arm.

Lung 7

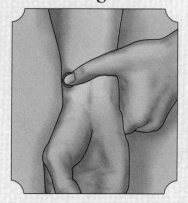

■ On the thumb side of the inner forearm, measure two finger widths above the crease in the wrist. Apply steady, firm pressure to the point site with your thumb, then repeat on the other arm.

Lung 10

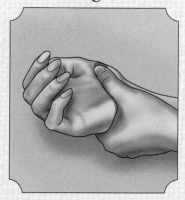

■ On the palm side of the hand, locate this point at the centre of the pad at the base of the thumb. Apply pressure with your other thumb while taking several deep breaths.

Gallery of Acupressure Techniques

Pericardium 3

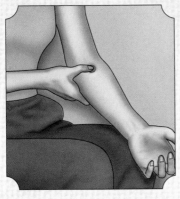

▓ Locate the point along the biceps tendon at the elbow crease, in a direct line with your ring finger. Use your thumb to apply firm pressure, then repeat on the other arm.

Pericardium 6

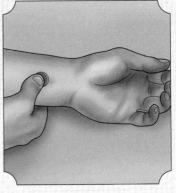

▓ To find this point, measure two finger widths above the centre of the wrist crease on the inside of your arm. With your thumb, press between the two bones of the forearm. Repeat on the other arm.

Small Intestine 3

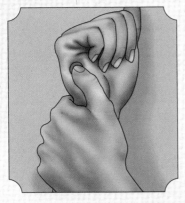

▓ Make a loose fist, then twist your wrist to view the side of your little finger. Using your thumb, apply pressure to the side of your palm just below the knuckle of the little finger, between the bone and muscle.

Small Intestine 17

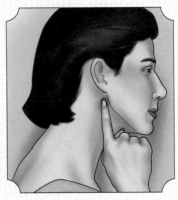

▓ Place your index fingers just below your earlobes, in the indentations at the back of the jawbone. Apply light pressure while breathing deeply.

CONTINUED

Spleen 3

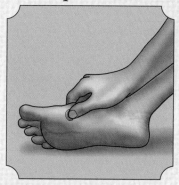

■ Locate the indentation on the inside of the foot, just behind the bulge made by the large joint of the big toe. Maintain steady pressure on the point site with your thumb. Repeat on the other foot.

Spleen 4

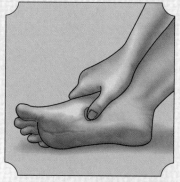

■ On the inside arch of your foot, measure one thumb width back from the ball of the foot. Apply pressure to this point with your thumb, and then repeat on the other foot.

Spleen 6

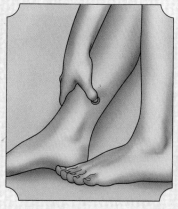

■ Measure four finger widths up from the top of the right inside anklebone. With your thumb, press near the edge of the shinbone. Repeat on the other leg. (Do not apply pressure to this point if you are pregnant.)

Spleen 8

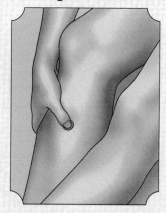

■ On the inside of the lower leg, locate the depression four finger widths below the knee. Press firmly between your calf muscle and your leg bone.

Gallery of Acupressure Techniques

Spleen 9

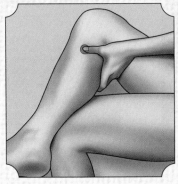

■ Place your thumb in the depression between the tibia and calf muscle on the inside of your leg, just below the knee joint. Press under the large bulge of the bone.

Spleen 10

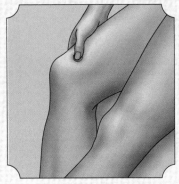

■ Bend your knee slightly to find this point, located two thumb widths up from the top of your knee, in line with the inner edge of the kneecap. Press on the bulge of the muscle with your thumb.

Spleen 12

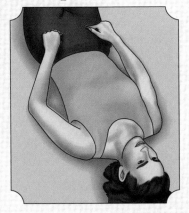

■ In the pelvic area, use your fingertips to press the middle of the crease where the leg joins the trunk of the body.

Stomach 2

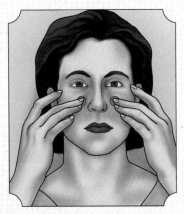

■ Measure one finger width below the lower ridge of the eye sockets, in line with the pupils. Press into the indentation of the cheeks.

CONTINUED

Gallery of Acupressure Techniques

Stomach 3

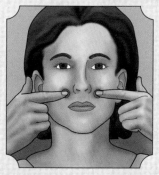

■ Place your index fingers at the bottom of your cheekbones, directly under the pupils of your eyes, then press firmly.

Stomach 7

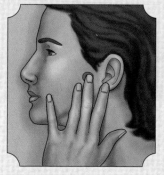

■ With your middle finger, feel on either side of your jaw one thumb width in front of your ears. Press the point site in the slight indentation along the upper jaw line.

Stomach 25

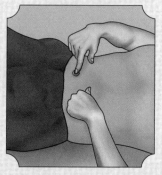

■ Place the index fingers of both hands two finger widths from your navel on either side. Press down firmly and breathe deeply.

Stomach 36

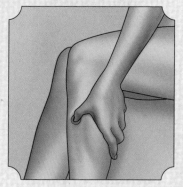

■ Measure four finger widths below the kneecap just outside the shinbone (flex your foot; you should feel a muscle bulge at the point site). Press the point steadily with a finger or thumb, then repeat on the other leg.

Stomach 44

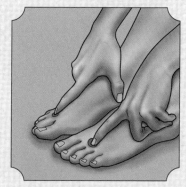

■ Using your index fingers, press lightly on the webbing between the second and third toes of each foot.

Gallery of Acupressure Techniques

Triple Warmer 3

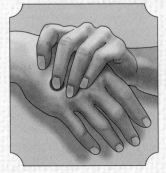

■ On the back of the hand, press firmly into the furrow just below the fourth and fifth knuckles (between the ring and little fingers). Repeat on the other hand.

Triple Warmer 5

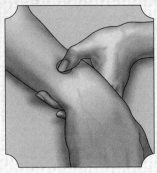

■ Centre your thumb on the top of your forearm, two thumb widths from the wrist joint, and press firmly. Repeat on the other arm.

Triple Warmer 6

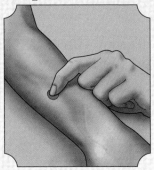

■ Measure about three finger widths from the wrist on the top of the forearm, then press this point with your thumb or index finger. Repeat on the other arm.

Triple Warmer 17

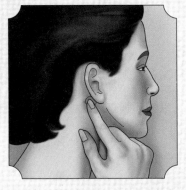

■ Using the tips of your index or middle fingers, find the hollows behind the earlobes where the ears meet the jawbone. Press lightly and breathe deeply.

Hiccup 1

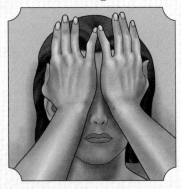

■ To stop hiccups, place your palms over both eyes, with heels resting on your cheekbones. Massage gently by pressing the pads below your thumbs towards your palms, then follow instructions for Governing Vessel 25.

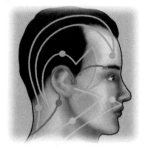

Target Ailments

- Arthritis
- Asthma
- Athletic Injuries
- Back Problems
- Bursitis
- Chronic Fatigue Syndrome
- Common Cold
- Depression
- Earache
- Gout
- Haemorrhoids
- Headache
- Indigestion
- Insomnia
- Nausea
- Pain, Chronic
- Sinusitis
- Sore Throat
- Stress
- Tendinitis
- Toothache

Acupuncture

T he healing technique of acupuncture, like other therapeutic approaches in the traditional practice of Chinese medicine (pages 45-48), is founded on the principle that internal harmony is essential for good health. Fundamental to this harmony is the concept of chi (sometimes spelled 'qi'), a vital energy or life force that ebbs and flows with changes in a person's mental, physical and spiritual well-being. Chi is said to circulate through the body within 14 invisible channels called meridians (see the illustrations on pages 24-25), forming a network called the web of life. A balanced, freely flowing chi is said to generate good health, while a sluggish, blocked or overstimulated chi is believed to cause illness. Acupuncturists strive to encourage proper chi circulation by manipulating it at 'chi gateways' just below the skin; the manipulation is achieved by inserting hair-thin needles at these gateways, which are more commonly known as acupoints. The stimulation that results is said to enable a person to achieve internal harmony, a state that allows the body's self-healing mechanisms to engage.

Origins

Acupuncture has been practised in China for about 4,500 years. Its spread to the West has been relatively slow but steady nonetheless. The first real surge in popularity came in the United States in 1971, following a story by a *New York Times* journalist who had been successfully treated for pain with acupuncture during a visit to China.

What It's Good For

Traditionally, acupuncturists have treated scores of different illnesses, as indicated by the list at left, which represents only a sampling of them. Although acupuncture's primary use in the West has been to alleviate pain, its therapeutic applications have been gradually expanding. Today, acupuncture is employed in treating addictions, controlling weight and enhancing recuperation following surgery or stroke.

Visiting a Professional

In order to properly evaluate your needs, during a first visit an acupuncturist will observe you closely, check your pulse, look at your tongue and ask many questions about your health and your lifestyle. These are customary diagnostic routines employed by practitioners of all forms of Chinese medicine.

Acupuncture

After this evaluation, the therapy itself can begin. Typically, the acupuncturist inserts acupuncture needles into the skin at the appropriate acupoints, then twirls them and, possibly, applies a gentle electric current (which is believed to enhance effectiveness). The needles may penetrate as little as a fraction of an inch (on the fingertips, for example) or as much as 3–4 in (7.5–10 cm), where a thick layer of fat or muscle exists. The procedure usually causes little pain, although patients often feel numbness where the needles are inserted, and perhaps a bit of tingling.

In addition to—or sometimes instead of—inserting needles, acupuncturists may opt for a treatment called moxibustion. This consists of applying heat directly above acupuncture points by means of small bundles of smouldering herbs, usually mugwort leaf. The practitioner may also employ acupressure *(pages 6-7)*.

Well-being

Because acupuncture's ultimate goal is to maximize the body's own healing abilities, it is little surprise that acupuncture treatments are considered helpful in maintaining as well as restoring health. Indeed, acupuncturists are trained to recognize so-called disharmonies early, often before they develop into full-blown disease.

What the Critics Say

An increasing number of conventional doctors are being trained in acupuncture and offering it to their patients. However, many others find it hard to accept acupuncture's invisible energy-path theory of effectiveness. The 'placebo effect' is most often cited as the reason acupuncture works—an argument that has not, however, held up to scientific testing. Some say that the pain of inserting acupuncture needles distracts the patient from his or her original pain, but this would not account for acupuncture's reputed success in treating other, painless ailments; also, properly inserted needles are not usually painful.

Research indicates that acupuncture stimulates the body to release its own natural painkillers (endorphins and encephalins), as well as an anti-inflammatory agent (cortisol). Whether enough of these natural chemicals are released to account for acupuncture's apparent success has yet to be determined. ■

CAUTION

While acupuncture can help manage the pain of labour and delivery, it is generally not recommended for other purposes during pregnancy because it may stimulate uterine contractions and could induce labour.

FOR MORE INFO

Following is a list of organizations you can contact to learn more about acupuncture:

British Acupuncture Council
63 Jeddo Road
London W12 9HQ
020 8735 0400
fax: 020 8735 0404

Institute for Complementary Medicine
PO Box 194
London SE16 1QZ
fax: 020 7237 5175

CONTINUED

✺ Meridians and Acupoints

*Chinese medicine teaches that energy flowing through invisible chan-
nels in the body called meridians may be manipulated by pressure (acupressure), the insertion of fine needles (acupuncture) or warmth (moxibustion) to treat disease and improve health. Meridians and related
acupoints are listed below. For more information, see the Gallery of Acupressure Techniques, pages 8-21.*

● Bladder
1 BL 1
2 BL 2
3 BL 7
4 BL 10
5 BL 13
6 BL 23
7 BL 25
8 BL 27
9 BL 28
10 BL 29
11 BL 30
12 BL 31
13 BL 32
14 BL 33
15 BL 34
16 BL 40
17 BL 57
18 BL 58
19 BL 60

● Conception Vessel
20 CV 4
21 CV 6
22 CV 12
23 CV 17
24 CV 22

● Gall Bladder
25 GB 2
26 GB 8
27 GB 14
28 GB 20
29 GB 21
30 GB 30
31 GB 34
32 GB 39
33 GB 40
34 GB 41

● Governing Vessel
35 GV 4
36 GV 14

37 GV 16
38 GV 20
39 GV 24.5
40 GV 25
41 GV 26

● Heart
42 HE 3
43 HE 7

● Kidney
44 KI 1
45 KI 2
46 KI 3
47 KI 5
48 KI 6
49 KI 7
50 KI 27

● Large Intestine
51 LI 4
52 LI 10
53 LI 11
54 LI 15
55 LI 20

● Liver
56 LV 2
57 LV 3
58 LV 8

● Lung
59 LU 1
60 LU 5
61 LU 6
62 LU 7
63 LU 9
64 LU 10

● Pericardium
65 PE 3
66 PE 6
67 PE 7

● Small Intestine
68 SI 3
69 SI 4
70 SI 5
71 SI 8
72 SI 10
73 SI 11
74 SI 17

● Spleen
75 SP 3
76 SP 4
77 SP 6
78 SP 8
79 SP 9
80 SP 10
81 SP 12
82 SP 16

● Stomach
83 ST 2
84 ST 3
85 ST 6
86 ST 7
87 ST 16
88 ST 18
89 ST 25
90 ST 35
91 ST 36
92 ST 40
93 ST 44

● Triple Warmer
94 TW 3
95 TW 4
96 TW 5
97 TW 15
98 TW 17
99 TW 21

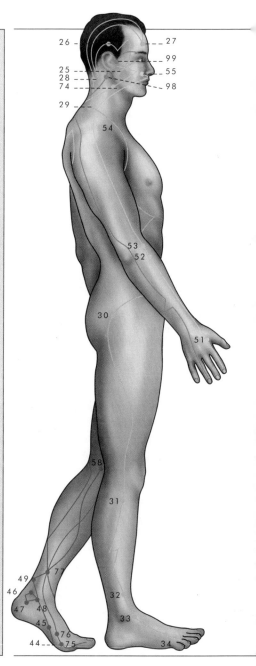

Acupuncture

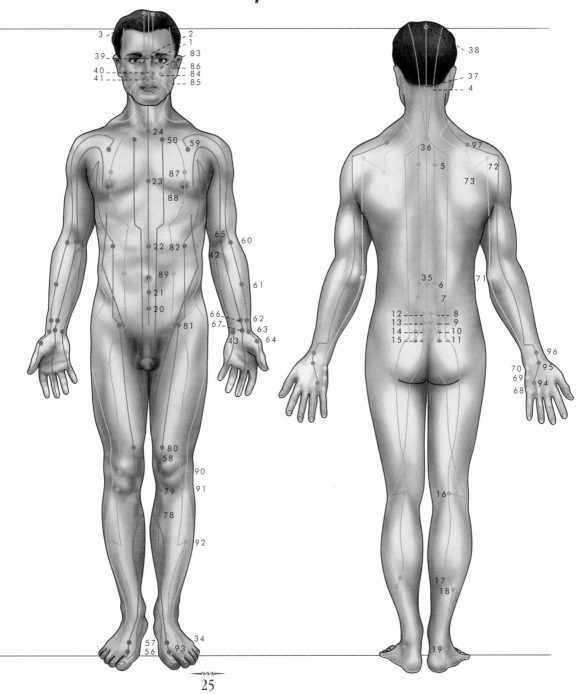

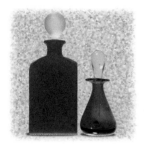

Target Ailments

- Bladder Infections
- Bronchitis
- Common Cold
- Conjunctivitis
- Depression
- Flu
- Immune Problems
- Indigestion
- Insomnia
- Laryngitis
- Menopause Problems
- Motion Sickness
- Muscle Cramps
- Nausea
- Sexually Transmitted Diseases
- Stress
- Tendinitis
- Tonsillitis
- Wind and Painful Wind
- Yeast Infections

$\mathcal{A}$romatherapy

romatherapy is the therapeutic use of essential oils—concentrated, fragrant extracts of plants—to promote relaxation and help relieve various symptoms. Suppliers of aromatherapy oils extract them from specific parts of plants—the roots, bark, stalks, flowers, leaves or fruit—by two methods: distillation uses successive evaporation and condensation to pull the oils from the plants; cold-pressing squeezes rinds or peels through a machine to press out the oils. Users then administer the oils in several ways, generally by applying them to the skin or inhaling their scents.

Some practitioners believe the oils have both physical and ethereal (spiritual) qualities and effects. They assert that the oils work on the emotions because the nerves involved in the sense of smell are directly linked to the brain's limbic system, which governs emotion, and that the active components of the oils give them specific therapeutic value, with antiseptic, antibacterial and antiviral effects common to many of them.

Origins

Ancient people used aromatic substances for medicinal, cosmetic and religious purposes. In the 10th century, the Arab doctor Avicenna described methods of distilling plants, although there is evidence that what came to be known as aromatherapy may have been known even in ancient times.

French chemist René-Maurice Gattefossé, who worked in a perfume factory, inaugurated the modern scientific use of essential oils in the 1920s and coined the term *aromatherapy*. After burning his hand in a chemical explosion, he quickly healed it without infection or scarring by applying lavender oil, which happened to be nearby. Gattefossé went on to classify the oils and their properties.

Aromatherapy gained widespread popularity in the United Kingdom and France in the 1980s, but it is less well known and researched in North America.

What It's Good For

Aromatherapists believe that all the oils affect the emotions in some way and that many also work on physical ailments. They think that as well as relieving stress, some oils may improve sluggish circulation, relieve pain, reduce swelling or cleanse the body of impurities. Others are used to treat bacterial or viral infections, burns, hypertension, arrhythmias, respiratory conditions, insomnia, depression and many other ailments.

Although patients with asthma may benefit from aromatherapy, they should use the oils only under a practitioner's supervision.

Aromatherapy

Preparations/Techniques

Essential oils may be applied externally and used in massage, or incorporated into compresses and ointments. They may also be inhaled or taken internally (orally, rectally or vaginally). Remember to follow all dilution, dosage and treatment guidelines as well as the cautions on the chart on the following pages.

A common aromatherapy technique is to dilute the oils in a vegetable carrier oil, such as safflower or sweet almond oil, for an aromatherapy massage. You can use basic massage strokes on yourself or a partner *(see the Gallery of Massage Techniques, pages 95-100)* to encourage relaxation or relieve specific problems. If you are prone to allergic reactions, test the oils first by putting a drop of oil on the inside of your elbow and waiting 24 hours for any reaction. During the massage, the skin absorbs the oil at the same time that the user inhales it.

Another way to use the oils is in an aromatic warm bath, which adds the therapeutic qualities of water to those of the oils. You may also apply hot or cold compresses, creams or lotions made from the oils directly to the skin. For respiratory conditions, insomnia, depression or stress, try breathing in the aromas using a steam inhaler or a fan-assisted apparatus. Remember to close your eyes when inhaling.

Buy oils from a reputable company and don't shop by price alone, because adulteration with chemicals and cheaper herbs is common. Consult a doctor before taking oils internally. Some oils, such as thuja, wormwood, mugwort leaf, tansy, hyssop, sage and eucalyptus, should never be taken internally.

Well-being

Essential oils are often incorporated into health programmes because they are easy and pleasant to use. Aromatherapists believe that regular use can re-establish balance and harmony within the body as well as soothe the mind and emotions.

What the Critics Say

Critics from conventional medicine point to the general lack of research in the field and to unscientific pronouncements of its proponents, such as references to ethereal effects and to the so-called subtle parts of the plants. Critics with a holistic viewpoint have faulted aromatherapy because the whole plant is not used. They note that chemical changes occur after a flower is cut that may adversely affect the therapeutic value of a given type of plant. ∎

CAUTION

Because the oils used in aromatherapy are available over the counter, some people may assume that they are all safe. However, they can have potentially serious side effects, including neurotoxicity and inducement of abortion, as well as skin reactions, allergies and liver damage. Overexposure to oils by inhalation can produce headache and fatigue. It's best to have a qualified aromatherapist supervise you when you use oils.

FOR MORE INFO

Following is an organization you can contact to learn more about aromatherapy:

Aromatherapy Organisations Council
PO Box 355
Croydon
Surrey CR9 2QP
020 8251 7912

CONTINUED

The 15 Most Effective Essential Oils

Name	Parts Used	Properties	Target Ailments
Bay laurel *Native to the Mediterranean, this hardy evergreen shrub or tree has dark green leaves and black berries. Its oil is greenish yellow and has a powerful spicy scent.*	●●● BERRIES DRIED LEAVES YOUNG TWIGS	An overall strengthener; can be an antiseptic, diuretic or sedative, and may help to expel wind and clear the lungs.	■ **Bay laurel** helps in digestive problems and appetite loss, relieves chronic bronchitis, colds, flu and tonsillitis, and treats scabies and lice. It also aids in rheumatic aches and pains and reduces swollen lymph nodes. CAUTION: Use in moderation. Avoid if pregnant.
Clary sage *This southern European plant has small blue or white flowers and large, hairy leaves. The oil is colourless or pale yellow-green and is used extensively in foods and drinks.*	FLOWERING TOPS LEAVES	A powerful, quick-acting relaxant; has warming effects; eases inflammation; anticonvulsive and antiseptic.	■ **Clary sage** soothes anxiety and stress, relieves menstrual and menopausal symptoms, and treats burns and eczema. CAUTION: Avoid during pregnancy or if you have high blood pressure. Do not drink alcohol while using.
Eucalyptus globulus *This native Australian evergreen is cultivated in several other areas, including California. The oil ranges from clear to yellow and has a penetrating smell.*	LEAVES TWIGS	Strongly antiseptic; antibacterial; expectorant; has stimulating, astringent and analgesic actions.	■ **Eucalyptus globulus** reduces fever; fights colds, flu, sinusitis and cough; helps relieve the symptoms of bronchitis; and is helpful in skin conditions such as boils and pimples. CAUTION: Do not take internally.
Everlasting *This strongly scented herb, with multi-branched stem and bright flowers, is native to the Mediterranean region and grows wild in the American Pacific North-west.*	FLOWERS FLOWERING TOPS	Anti-inflammatory and painkilling properties; prevents internal haemorrhage and swelling after injury.	■ **Everlasting** is effective in skin conditions such as scarring, sunburn and wounds. It relieves congestion of the liver or spleen, helps in bronchitis and flu, and is used to treat tendinitis, arthritic pain, and muscle aches, sprains and strains.
German chamomile *Native to Europe and Asia, this widely cultivated aromatic herb has feathery leaves and white flowers, and produces an inky blue strong-scented oil.*	FLOWERS	Anti-inflammatory, sedative, and pain-killing properties; also anti-allergic and antiseptic.	■ **German chamomile** alleviates digestive upsets, menstrual and menopausal problems, inflamed skin, burns, acne, boils, sunburn and cuts. It aids in arthritis and muscular pain, and helps to relieve symptoms of hay fever and bronchitis.
Lavender *Native to the Mediterranean, this evergreen shrub is now grown worldwide. You may release its familiar aroma by rubbing a flower or leaf between the fingers. The oil is clear or yellow-green.*	FLOWERING TOPS	Known for its calming, soothing and balancing effects; also has analgesic and antiseptic properties.	■ **Lavender** relieves headache, depression, insomnia, stress, muscular aches and sprains, menstrual pain and nausea. It also soothes skin conditions such as cuts, wounds, insect bites, burns and athlete's foot.
Lemon-scented eucalyptus *This tall evergreen, sometimes called a gum tree, is native to Australia. Its colourless or pale yellow oil has long been used for sachets in airing cupboards.*	LEAVES TWIGS	Sedative, anti-inflammatory, anti-septic and deodorant action; can kill bacteria, viruses and fungi.	■ **Lemon-scented eucalyptus** soothes mosquito bites and skin irritations. It also helps athlete's foot and herpes sores and relieves muscle tension and stress. CAUTION: Do not take internally.

Aromatherapy

Name	Parts Used	Properties	Target Ailments
Niaouli *Principally from Australia, this evergreen has a spongy bark and white flowers. The yellow or greenish oil has a camphorous odour and is found in health aids such as toothpaste.*	LEAVES YOUNG TWIGS	Antiseptic, analgesic and anti-allergic properties, as well as tissue-stimulating action helpful for healing.	**Niaouli** combats allergies, bronchitis, colds and flu; cleans minor wounds and burns; aids in acne, boils and insect bites; and helps relieve muscle aches and pains as well as toothache. It may also be used to treat bladder infection.
Palmarosa *Native to India and Pakistan, this wild tropical grass has a long stem and aromatic leaves. The oil is pale yellow or olive in colour, with a sweet floral scent.*	FLOWERS LEAVES	Antiviral, antibacterial and anti-septic properties, as well as an overall strengthening effect.	**Palmarosa** is diluted with almond oil to treat skin conditions such as cuts and wounds, acne, dermatitis, cold sores and scars. It also relieves symptoms of flu, fights intestinal and other infections and is helpful in stress-related conditions.
Peppermint *This perennial herb native to Europe and western Asia is cultivated around the world. Its oil is colourless, pale yellow or green and is a popular flavouring agent.*	FLOWERING TOPS LEAVES	Produces a warming effect (after an initial cooling action) and can relieve pain; also stimulates the liver.	**Peppermint** relieves indigestion, nausea and headache. It is helpful for neuralgia and muscle pain, and can aid in bronchitis, sinusitis and motion sickness. CAUTION: Use in moderation. Do not give to children under 30 months of age.
Rosemary *This Mediterranean evergreen shrub has silvery green leaves and pale blue flowers. The oil is colourless to pale yellow-green; its scent is minty in oils of good quality.*	FLOWERING TOPS LEAVES	A stimulant that invigorates the whole body and helps eliminate toxins; antiseptic and diuretic properties.	**Rosemary** is effective for indigestion, wind and liver problems. It fights bronchitis and flu, reduces fluid retention and helps treat depression. CAUTION: Avoid during pregnancy or if you have epilepsy or high blood pressure.
Tarragon *This bushy perennial plant native to Asia and Europe has narrow green leaves and small flowers. The colourless oil has an aroma similar to anise and is a popular food seasoning.*	LEAVES	Antispasmodic, diuretic and mild laxative properties; stimulant.	**Tarragon** helps with menstrual and menopausal symptoms and with digestive ailments such as wind, indigestion, hiccups and loss of appetite. It can aid in stress-related problems and in overcoming shock. CAUTION: Avoid during pregnancy.
Tea tree *Native to New South Wales, Australia, the tea tree or shrub has small, narrow leaves and yellow or purple flowers. Its tart oil ranges from colourless to pale yellow-green.*	LEAVES TWIGS	Antiseptic action against bacteria, fungi and viruses; soothing to the skin and mucous membranes.	**Tea tree** fights colds, flu, tonsillitis, bronchitis and sinusitis, and can treat skin ailments such as abscesses, acne and burns. It also helps clear vaginal thrush, vaginitis and bladder infections, and helps control *Candida* infection.
Thyme *This evergreen shrub native to the Mediterranean area has grey-green leaves and clusters of purple or white flowers. The oil's natural colour varies from red- or orange-brown to yellow.*	FLOWERING TOPS LEAVES	Strongly stimulating, antiseptic and antibacterial properties; also has antispasmodic and digestive actions.	**Thyme** helps in laryngitis and coughs and fights skin, bladder and other infections. It relieves joint pain, treats diarrhoea and wind and can help to expel intestinal worms. CAUTION: Avoid during pregnancy or if you have high blood pressure.
Ylang-ylang *Native to the Philippines, ylang-ylang is a tall tropical tree with large, fragrant flowers. The clear or yellow oil, used in perfumes and soaps, has a sweet, spicy aroma.*	FRESH FLOWERS	Both stimulant and sedative properties; also can regulate heart action.	**Ylang-ylang** helps with acne and oily skin and aids in depression, insomnia, impotence and other stress-related disorders. It can be a backup therapy for high blood pressure. CAUTION: Overuse can cause headache or nausea.

Target Ailments

- Allergies
- Angina
- Arthritis
- Cancer
- Cholesterol Problems
- Chronic Fatigue Syndrome
- Common Cold
- Constipation
- Depression
- Diabetes
- Diarrhoea
- Flu
- Headache
- Heartburn
- High Blood Pressure
- Immune Problems
- Insomnia
- Irritable Bowel Syndrome
- Premenstrual Syndrome
- Wind and Painful Wind

Ayurvedic Medicine

A yurvedic medicine is a system of diagnosis and treatment that has been practised in India for more than 2,500 years. The term 'ayurveda' comes from the Sanskrit roots āyuh, which means longevity, and veda, meaning knowledge. Ayurvedic theory holds that the human body represents the entire universe in microcosmic form, and that we come to know how we function as organisms only by observing and understanding the world around us. The key to health is maintaining a balance between the microcosmic body and the macrocosmic world, a relationship that is expressed in the concept of three physiological principles called doshas. The role of the Ayurvedic physician is to restore and maintain, through different types of therapies, diet, lifestyle and natural medicines, the balance of the three doshas that is appropriate for a given individual.

The Three Doshas

According to Ayurvedic theory, every person contains some amount of the universe's five basic elements: earth, air, fire, water and aether (or space). To describe and understand the combination of these elements that makes up each unique individual—and thereby to gain insights into aspects of personality as well as of physiology—Ayurvedic healers rely on the concept of *doshas*.

Doshas are general categories; each dosha consists of one or more of the universe's five basic elements. Ayurvedic practitioners recognize three main types of dosha: *vata, pitta* and *kapha*. Together these are called the *tridosha*.

Vata, 'wind', is a combination of aether (space) and air. As such, vata is associated with lightness and dispersion, and this concept encompasses both the movement of fluids and cells through the body and the flow of thoughts through the mind. According to Ayurvedic principles, people who are strongly influenced by vata are said to be active and often restless. Creative people often have a strong vata component in their makeup.

Pitta, 'bile', is composed of fire (some descriptions also mention water). The key to this dosha is the concept of transformation—apparent in such physical processes as the digestion of food to produce energy. Pitta is said to be the controlling force behind all of the body's metabolic activities. Persons primarily influenced by pitta are thought to be doers, in the sense of being quick to change things as needs arise. They also may be extremely competitive or aggressive.

Kapha, 'phlegm', is made up of earth and water elements. Structure is integral to kapha, as this dosha is said to provide the body's physical strength, stability and wound-healing abilities. A predominantly kapha person might be relatively heavy

Ayurvedic Medicine

and muscular, and would be likely to be characterized as having a stable and tranquil personality.

Doshic Balance

A given individual's natural constitution—known in Ayurvedic medicine as that person's *prakriti*—is a unique balance of the three doshas. Each person's prakriti is said to be present at the moment of conception. While every prakriti contains a certain amount of vata, pitta and kapha, one dosha usually predominates. According to Ayurveda, your prakriti not only describes your constitution but also regulates your physical, emotional and mental processes. By living a lifestyle that conforms to your specific prakriti, you can achieve optimum health. If, however, in the course of your daily life you subject yourself to overeating, stress, inadequate or excessive sleep or other similar conditions, you can excite one or more of the doshas, causing a disruption of your doshic balance (and therefore your prakriti), which is virtually guaranteed to lead to illness.

Ayurvedic practitioners advocate diets and lifestyles that reinforce the doshic balance, and encourage close vigilance (through body and mind-awareness techniques such as meditation) to identify imbalances. When an imbalance is detected and confirmed by an Ayurvedic practitioner, immediate corrective measures are prescribed using Ayurvedic therapies and remedies.

Origins

Historical evidence suggests that the medical system we now call Ayurveda began in India around the sixth century BC, coinciding roughly with the lifetime of the Buddha (although some scholars contend that it began much earlier). According to tradition, holy men, or *rishis,* gathered together in a hermitage high in the Himalayas to compile the healing wisdom they had attained via divine inspiration. Their medical knowledge was then transmitted to the people as part of the sacred Hindu scriptures known as the Vedas. The rishis intended that Ayurveda would maximize the health of the body and the mind, and that this would create an unencumbered path to a person's spiritual fulfilment.

Through the centuries, Ayurvedic philosophy has spread worldwide. In the last few hundred years, foreign influence in India has overshadowed much traditional knowledge, including Ayurveda. The last 35 years or so, however, have witnessed a powerful resurgence in interest, among both practitioners and patients. In India today, Ayurveda is now a popular—though not exclusive—choice for almost 80 per cent of the population; conventional Western-style allopathic medicine, homoeopathy, Arabic Unani medicine and Siddha medicine, in the south, are also commonly practised.

CAUTION

Some Ayurvedic preparations contain harmful substances such as lead, mercury and arsenic. Although these substances may be described as 'inactivated' and therefore safe, their safety has not been proved. Avoid all preparations containing even minute amounts of heavy metals or dangerous chemicals. Ayurvedic medicine is a comprehensive system of healthcare; however, it is not always appropriate for treating serious injuries or problems that require surgery.

CONTINUED

Ayurvedic Medicine CONTINUED

Ayurveda is steadily growing in popularity in the West, where two types of Ayurvedic medicine co-exist: traditional Ayurveda and Maharishi Ayur-Veda. Traditional Ayurveda is based on the ancient textbooks of the master physicians Caraka, Sushruta and Vagbhata. Many traditional practitioners have been trained in India's Ayurveda colleges, but the Ayurvedic Medical Association UK does run a part-time diploma course.

Maharishi Ayur-Veda is a modern effort by Maharishi Mahesh Yogi (the Indian teacher who introduced transcendental meditation to the West in the 1960s) to blend traditional Ayurvedic medicine with transcendental meditation. Maharishi Ayur-Veda practitioners are trained in North America, and this is the more popular type of Ayurvedic medicine in the United States. (Maharishi Ayur-Veda is also the name of a company that sells Ayurvedic products and services.)

What It's Good For

While its primary focus is preventive, Ayurveda also encompasses healing remedies for hundreds of ailments. Practitioners especially recommend Ayurvedic therapies for the relief of chronic, metabolic and stress-related problems. Numerous studies are under way to determine if Ayurvedic remedies may inhibit breast cancer; increase mobility and reduce the pain of arthritis; allay chemotherapy's side effects; hasten recuperation following conventional surgery; decrease serum cholesterol; alleviate symptoms of Parkinson's disease; reduce insulin dependence for diabetics; and assist in recovery from heroin addiction.

Two Forms of Treatment

Ayurvedic practitioners use many preparations and techniques, including hatha-yoga *(see Yoga, pages 141-142),* sounds, scents, foods, spices, colours, minerals, medicines and gems. These can be separated into two basic types of Ayurvedic treatment: constitutional and therapeutic.

Constitutional treatments encompass adjustments in lifestyle and the taking of preparations that are believed to enhance and preserve good health. These preventive measures might include engaging in *pranayama,* or breathing exercises; readjusting your sleeping and eating schedules to correspond with your prakriti; performing Ayurvedic massage (called *abhyanga*) to re-establish your energy flow, or *prana;* or taking regular herbal supplements called *rasayanas* to cleanse your body and harmonize your prakriti. The principal form of constitutional treatment is known as *panchakarma,* and it can last anywhere from three days to three weeks. It is an intensive and individualized five-step cleansing process that incorporates a special diet and various massages, herbal treatments and evacuation procedures, all with the goal of purifying the body and the mind.

Ayurvedic Medicine

Therapeutic treatments are specific healing regimens. According to Ayurvedic theory, all disease originates in the gastrointestinal tract, and is ultimately caused by decreased enzyme activity and poor digestion. Improperly digested foods are said to form a sludge-like substance called *ama* that blocks the body's digestive and energy channels. Practitioners use therapeutic treatments (called *anamaya*) to fight disease by ridding the body of ama and re-establishing a balanced prakriti. These treatments might include medicinal remedies (selected from some 8,000 herbal, mineral, fruit and vegetable preparations used in Ayurvedic practice); cleansing procedures such as therapeutic vomiting (inducing vomiting to expel toxins) or herbal enemas; and bloodletting, which is believed to detoxify the blood.

Dietary change is by far the most common form of constitutional and therapeutic treatment. Certain foods are credited with the ability to strengthen or weaken the doshas, and practitioners often suggest specific diets to help re-establish a patient's prakriti.

OF SPECIAL INTEREST

Healing Elements

Using medicinal herbs and prescribing nutritional changes are not the only healing techniques espoused by Ayurvedic practitioners. Colours, aromas, gems and stones are also believed to activate the body's healing potential. When worn or held close to the body, certain stones and gems are said to release their healing energy and engage the body's own energy centres. Aromas are said to help soothe the mind—a belief shared by practitioners of aromatherapy (pages 26-27)—and to pacify disturbed doshas. The seven colours of the rainbow are believed to be related to the tridosha, and therefore to be helpful in balancing the prakriti. To take advantage of colour therapy, practitioners may advise patients to drink water from a glass wrapped in coloured paper. The colour's power is said to infuse the water and be transported to the person who drinks it.

Visiting a Professional

Ayurveda dictates that every person is responsible for his or her own health. This is not to negate the value of the practitioner-patient relationship, however. Although Ayurvedic preparations are available to everyone, it is difficult (if not impossible) to identify what you need without a practitioner's help. And when illness strikes, a practitioner's advice is essential.

Expect your first visit with your *vaidya*, or Ayurvedic doctor, to last 45 to 90 minutes. In determining your unique tridosha and prakriti, he or she will ask questions about your emotional, spiritual and physical health, your diet and your lifestyle. You may also be asked to complete a written questionnaire that delves further into your physical and spiritual health.

Your vaidya will check your pulse to help establish your prakriti and determine your overall condition; rates,

CONTINUED

intensities and rhythms of an individual's pulse are believed to indicate specific physical, mental and metabolic conditions. The practitioner will observe you closely, paying particular attention to the condition of your tongue, skin, lips, eyes and nails. Some practitioners also rely on laboratory analysis of blood, urine and stools to help in diagnosing your prakriti.

After determining your constitution, your vaidya will use an integrative approach to consider your specific physical, emotional, mental and spiritual needs, and recommend treatments to harmonize your lifestyle with your prakriti.

Well-being

Preventive medicine is the central tenet of Ayurvedic healing. According to Ayurveda, health is achieved and maintained by first identifying a person's prakriti and then assigning the proper constitutional or therapeutic remedies to maintain his or her doshic balance. Practitioners encourage their patients to stay in close contact, so that therapies and regimens may be adjusted as needed.

What the Critics Say

Ayurveda's use of non-standard techniques of diagnosis and treatment and its reliance on organic medicines tend to make conventional Western physicians and scientists uneasy. But not all conventional physicians oppose Ayurveda. Some doctors have received introductory Ayurvedic training and use Ayurveda to complement their conventional-style practices. As Ayurveda's popularity continues to increase within the general population, this trend is likely to continue.

Some criticism of Ayurveda is directed specifically towards the Maharishi Ayur-Veda system. Detractors allege that the promoters of Maharishi Ayur-Veda may be more interested in selling medicine than in healing. Some insist that descriptions of Maharishi Ayur-Veda's power and potential have been wildly exaggerated. Others question whether Maharishi Ayur-Veda represents authentic Ayurvedic science. Still, Maharishi Ayur-Veda remains the most popular form of Ayurvedic medicine in the United States. Both traditional Ayurveda and Maharishi Ayur-Veda therapies are currently being investigated in scientific laboratories around the world. ∎

FOR MORE INFO

Following is an organization you can contact to learn more about Ayurvedic medicine:

Ayurvedic Medical Association UK
59 Dulverton Road
South Croydon
Surrey CR2 8PJ
0850 670 706
fax: 020 8333 7904

$\mathcal{B}$ody Work

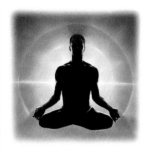

Body work is an umbrella term for the many techniques that promote relaxation and treat ailments (especially those of the musculoskeletal system) through lessons in proper movement and posture, exercise, massage and various other forms of bodily manipulation. These techniques can be divided into three broad categories—massage, movement awareness and structural realignment, and energy balancing—although the majority include more than one of these elements. Most take a holistic view of health and emphasize treatment of the mind as well as of the body. Sceptics point out, however, that therapeutic claims made for these techniques are usually based on anecdotal observation rather than on controlled scientific studies.

Some of the many body-work techniques are explored in detail below and on the following pages. Massage, which is generally considered a form of body work, is described separately on pages 92-94.

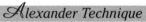
Alexander Technique

This form of body work was developed in the late 1800s by an Australian Shakespearean actor named Frederick Matthias Alexander, whose voice often became hoarse during performances, jeopardizing his career. When the rest and medication prescribed by his physician failed to provide a reliable cure, Alexander decided to find out for himself the cause of his vocal problem. Using a mirror, he studied the way he spoke and concluded that he was unconsciously tensing his body in a way that was interfering with the correct relationship between his head, neck and back—and that this tension was affecting his voice. In the course of finding a way to correct this damaging habit, Alexander developed the muscle-releasing and postural technique that bears his name. Although he cured his propensity to hoarseness and returned to the stage, Alexander eventually left acting—and Australia—to teach his technique to others in England and America.

What It's Good For • The Alexander technique teaches people how to release painful muscle tension, improve posture and move with greater ease. Old, damaging habits of sitting, moving and speaking are replaced with new, more efficient ones. People who practise the technique find it reduces stress and fatigue.

Target Ailments

- Arthritis
- Athletic Injuries
- Back Problems
- Bursitis
- Pain, Chronic
- Tendinitis

CONTINUED

Body Work CONTINUED

CAUTION

You should avoid body work that involves massage if you have an open wound, a bone fracture or dislocation, an infectious disease, a contagious skin condition, severe varicose veins or any heart problem. Some health professionals are concerned that the deep massage associated with some of these techniques may cause existing cancer cells to metastasize, or spread, in the body. If you have cancer, you may want to ask your body-work practitioner to consult with your consultant before undergoing one of these techniques.

FOR MORE INFO

Contact the following organization to learn more about the Alexander technique:

Society of Teachers of the Alexander Technique
020 7351 0828

Because it improves postural habits, the Alexander technique can also help relieve back, knee and other pain caused by the improper use of muscles; it is especially helpful for disc problems and sciatica. The technique has also been effective in relieving the discomfort associated with arthritis, bursitis and other conditions involving muscles and joints.

Preparations/Techniques • The Alexander technique is traditionally taught in one-on-one lessons, although some instructors also offer group classes. Basic to the technique is learning how to release your neck muscles so that your head can balance freely on top of your neck. This, in turn, allows your back to lengthen, eliminating compression in the spine.

During a lesson, the teacher will analyse the way you sit, stand, walk and bend. He or she will then use verbal instructions and gentle touch to guide you into releasing muscle tension, improving posture and moving with more freedom. You will learn to apply this improved use of your body to everyday tasks, from sitting in a chair to carrying packages to talking on the phone. The Alexander technique does not involve exercises. However, you will learn to apply it to any sport or exercise programme you do on a regular basis. Advocates believe this will help you avoid injury and also increase the benefit you receive from your regular exercise programme.

Lessons in the Alexander technique generally last 30 to 45 minutes. Wear loose, non-restrictive clothing. Your instructor will work with you while you are lying on a table and also while you are moving about.

Well-being • Practitioners of this technique believe it promotes health by helping people learn how to move within their physical environment in a relaxed and efficient manner that promotes healthy mental and physical functioning.

What the Critics Say
Although correcting poor posture has been known to help prevent back and neck pain, the specific therapeutic benefits of the Alexander technique have not been demonstrated in controlled scientific studies. One study has shown that the technique can be beneficial to healthy adults by enabling them to breathe more efficiently, but it involved only a small number of participants.

Body Work

Aston-Patterning

Target Ailments

▦ Athletic Injuries

▦ Back Problems

▦ Stress

This type of body work was developed in the 1970s by a California dancer named Judith Aston. A decade earlier, two separate car accidents had left her with a disabling back injury. At a doctor's suggestion, Aston went to see Ida Rolf, whose unique form of deep massage and postural retraining known as Rolfing (page 42) helped Aston regain full body movement. Aston began working with Rolf to develop a movement maintenance programme that would help people sustain structural changes brought about by Rolfing. She eventually broke away from Rolfing to develop and teach her own form of body work.

What It's Good For • Practitioners claim it can help relieve acute or chronic pain such as that caused by poor posture or muscle tension. They also believe it can improve balance, increase strength and endurance and relieve fatigue. The goal is to help people find more comfortable and efficient ways to work, play and rest.

Preparations/Techniques • Aston-Patterning is generally taught in one-on-one sessions with a trained practitioner. Each session can last from one to two hours and may include any or all of the following components: movement education, or neurokinetics, which involves learning how to decrease body tension and move more efficiently; three types of body work that release tensions held in different body structures; ergonomic training, which teaches how to modify home and work environments in ways that encourage good posture and efficient movement; and fitness training, which helps to stretch, loosen and tone muscles throughout the body.

Well-being • Like most alternative therapies, Aston-Patterning focuses on promoting health and well-being—goals it seeks to achieve by improving how the body moves and functions.

What the Critics Say
Critics note that Aston-Patterning's therapeutic effectiveness has not been demonstrated in controlled studies.

FOR MORE INFO
Contact the following organization
to learn more about
Aston-Patterning:

The Aston Training Center
PO Box 3568
Incline Village, NV 89450
USA

CONTINUED

Body Work CONTINUED

Target Ailments

■ Back Problems

■ Insomnia

■ Multiple Sclerosis

■ Pain, Chronic

■ Stress

Feldenkrais Method

This body-work technique was developed by Moshe Feldenkrais, a Russian-born Israeli physicist who became interested in the physics of body movement during the 1940s, after experiencing a disabling knee injury. He drew on the earlier work of Frederick Matthias Alexander (pages 35-36)—as well as on his own intense study of anatomy, biochemistry, neurophysiology and other sciences related to human movement—to create this system for improving posture, movement and breathing.

What It's Good For • Feldenkrais practitioners claim the method can help people with chronic musculoskeletal problems, such as back or knee pain. They also report success helping people overcome some of the physical limitations brought on by an injury or by a chronic medical condition, such as cerebral palsy or multiple sclerosis. Other benefits cited include improved digestion, more restful sleep, greater mental alertness, increased energy and reduced stress.

Preparations/Techniques • The Feldenkrais method teaches how to recognize and then break improper habits of movement. You can learn the technique through a group class or one-on-one lessons. In group classes a practitioner verbally guides students through a sequence of movements designed to teach how to relax and abandon habitual patterns of movement that reveal unconscious tension. Private lessons provide similar guidance, although here the practitioner also uses slow, gentle touch to help you feel exactly where and how your body is tensing and moving incorrectly. Both types of sessions last about 45 minutes to an hour. You'll also learn exercises to practise at home.

Well-being • Feldenkrais practitioners believe that by helping people release unnecessary muscle tension and move in a freer and more graceful way, injuries and stress-related illness can be prevented.

What the Critics Say

The small amount of objective research that has been done on the therapeutic benefits of the Feldenkrais method has been inconclusive.

FOR MORE INFO

Contact the following organization to learn more about the Feldenkrais method:

The Feldenkrais Guild
PO Box 370
London N10 3XA
07000 785 506

Body Work

Hellerwork

Hellerwork was developed by Joseph Heller, a former aerospace engineer who began studying with Ida Rolf in the early 1970s. At the time, Rolfing (page 42) did not include movement education, which Heller thought essential for helping people break old, destructive movement patterns. Nor did it include an exploration of the psychological dynamics behind such habits, which Heller believed was also necessary to root out tension. So in 1978 Heller founded his own method, which includes deep massage, movement education and therapeutic discussion.

What It's Good For • Hellerwork is based on the premise that a misaligned body limits movement and flexibility, leading to fatigue, physical deterioration and premature ageing. By realigning the body, Hellerwork is thought to release chronic tension and increase flexibility, which in turn reduces stress, increases energy and creates an overall feeling of youthfulness.

Preparations/Techniques • The Hellerwork programme consists of eleven 90-minute private sessions, each with a theme, such as 'reaching out', and concentrating on a different part of the body. Each session begins with a deep connective-tissue massage to reduce body tension and realign the musculoskeletal system. Movement lessons follow on how to sit, stand, bend and walk with more fluidity and balance. The practitioner will also ask about emotional patterns that may have led to physical tension. You may be asked, for example, about how easy or difficult it is for you to be assertive or to reach out to others. The therapy, however, does not require you to answer any questions that you find too painful or uncomfortable.

Well-being • Practitioners believe Hellerwork promotes wellness by breaking the muscular rigidity caused by unconscious habits, so people can better align themselves with gravity and move with more ease and energy.

What the Critics Say
The therapeutic benefits of this particular technique have not been demonstrated in controlled studies.

Target Ailments

- Athletic Injuries
- Back Problems
- Carpal Tunnel Syndrome
- Stress

FOR MORE INFO
Contact the following organization to learn more about Hellerwork:

European Hellerwork Association
36 Langley Hill
Kings Langley
Herts. WD4 9HE
020 7723 5676

website: www.hellerwork.co.uk
email: roger@golten.net

CONTINUED

Body Work CONTINUED

Target Ailments

- Arthritis
- Athletic Injuries
- Back Problems
- Carpal Tunnel Syndrome
- Headache
- Menstrual Problems
- Multiple Sclerosis
- TMJ Syndrome

Myotherapy

The term 'myotherapy' is used here to refer specifically to the technique known formally as Bonnie Prudden Myotherapy. It is an offshoot of trigger point injection therapy, a medical treatment developed in the 1940s that involved injecting saline and the drug procaine directly into painful muscles, or 'trigger points', to get them to relax. In 1976 physical fitness pioneer Bonnie Prudden discovered that the injections were unnecessary, as simple manual pressure on the trigger points could produce similar results. This finding led to the development of her form of myotherapy—a deep-pressure massage used to reduce tension and pain originating in specific points in the muscle layers of the body.

What It's Good For • Practitioners claim this therapy is beneficial for a variety of muscle-related conditions, including back, shoulder and neck pain; headaches; repetitive motion injuries; menstrual cramps; sports injuries; and TMJ syndrome. They say it can also help relieve pain associated with such diseases as arthritis, multiple sclerosis and lupus. Practitioners emphasize, however, that myotherapy does not cure disease, but rather helps relieve pain and ease recovery.

Preparations/Techniques • Sessions last about an hour. The therapist will ask questions about your sports activities, occupation, injuries and illnesses, and will test your muscles' strength and flexibility. Then, using fingers, knuckles, and elbows, the therapist will apply pressure to trigger points—those areas in your muscles that the therapist believes are responsible for your pain. Treatment is followed by passive stretching of affected muscles. You will be given corrective exercises to do at home to help keep your muscles free of spasms and pain.

Well-being • Myotherapists believe that by reducing pain and helping to restore the body's full range of motion, they can improve an individual's overall health and sense of well-being.

What the Critics Say
Critics point out that massaging trigger points is not unique to this therapy alone.

FOR MORE INFO
Contact the following organization to learn more about myotherapy:

Bonnie Prudden Pain Erasure
7800 East Speedway Boulevard
Tucson, AZ 85710
USA

Body Work

Reiki

Reiki (pronounced ray-key) practitioners claim this ancient form of healing originated in Tibet thousands of years ago and was rediscovered in the mid-1800s by Mikao Usui, an educator at a Christian seminary in Kyoto, Japan. According to Reiki tradition, Usui spent 21 days fasting on a sacred mountain outside Kyoto, where he experienced a vision that revealed how the universal life energy described in ancient Sanskrit writings could be activated through a hands-on approach to healing. Usui named this healing method Reiki, after the healing aspect of the energy.

What It's Good For • Reiki is used to treat a wide variety of conditions, from minor ailments such as heartburn to chronic diseases such as arthritis.

Preparations/Techniques • Only a trained practitioner may administer Reiki. During a healing session, the practitioner will gently lay his or her hands over the chakras, or energy centres, of your body to enable healing energy to flow more fully into your body. Treatments last from 30 to 60 minutes and are usually carried out in four sessions over four successive days. For some conditions, people receive treatments once a week for one or two months. You will be instructed to drink substantial quantities of water and herbal tea during the treatment period to help cleanse your body of toxins. You may be told to avoid stimulants, such as coffee and white sugar, which can interfere with the cleansing process.

Well-being • Reiki practitioners believe the body becomes ill when the universal life energy is out of balance. Thus, by bringing balance and harmony to the body, Reiki enables the body and the mind to heal and remain healthy.

What the Critics Say

Evidence of Reiki's benefits is mainly anecdotal; very few controlled studies of it have been done. Because Reiki is often used to treat illnesses, critics worry that seriously ill patients will not receive the conventional medical care they need. Competent Reiki practitioners, however, do not discourage their patients from receiving such care.

Target Ailments

- Arthritis
- Athletic Injuries
- Chronic Fatigue Syndrome
- Heartburn
- Indigestion
- Insomnia
- Irritable Bowel Syndrome
- Pain, Chronic
- Stress

FOR MORE INFO

Following is an organization you can contact to learn more about Reiki:

The Kevala Centre
Hunsdon Road
Torquay
Devon TQ1 1QB
01803 215678
email:
information@kevala.co.uk
website: www.kevala.co.uk

CONTINUED

Body Work CONTINUED

Target Ailments

- Athletic Injuries
- Back Problems
- Carpal Tunnel Syndrome
- Stress

Rolfing

This form of body work was developed in the 1940s and 1950s by Ida Rolf, a biochemist who wanted to improve the health of her friends and family and cure her own spinal curvature problem. After much study she decided that many physical and mental problems are caused by the body being out of alignment with gravity. She felt that by deeply massaging the fascia—the connective tissue enclosing muscles—most bodies could be brought back into alignment. This deep massage was called structural integration, but it became better known by its trademarked name, Rolfing.

What It's Good For • Rolfing is said to ease chronic pain and stiffness, especially that caused by poor posture. Many athletes, dancers, musicians and others seeking to improve physical performance in their professions and daily activities say they have been helped by Rolfing. Rolfers also claim the technique can help ease anxiety caused by chronic stress.

Preparations/Techniques • Rolfing is usually applied in 10 one-hour sessions. In each session, a specific area is massaged, or 'manipulated'. Rolfers use their fingers, knuckles and elbows during the sometimes painful manipulations. The intent is to loosen adhesions in the fascia and bring the head, shoulders, thorax, pelvis and legs into improved alignment with gravity. In a separate programme, patients are instructed on how to move their body in more efficient ways.

Well-being • Rolfers believe that stretching and lengthening the fascia, and thus bringing the body into proper alignment with gravity, helps keep the body in a state that is free of stress.

What the Critics Say

Critics point out that no large, controlled studies of Rolfing have been carried out. One study of 10 cerebral palsy patients had mixed results. Critics are also concerned that some Rolfers use the technique to treat depression and other psychological disorders but are not qualified to do so.

FOR MORE INFO

Contact the following organization to learn more about Rolfing:

The Rolf Institute
205 Canyon Boulevard
Boulder, CO 80306
USA
e-mail: Rolf Inst@aol.com

Body Work

Therapeutic Touch

During the 1970s Dolores Krieger, a nursing professor at New York University, brought together a variety of ancient 'hands-on' healing practices into a modern technique she called therapeutic touch. Like many of its older predecessors, therapeutic touch is based on the premise that disease reflects a blockage in the flow of energy that surrounds and permeates the body. Krieger devised a four-step process by which a therapeutic touch practitioner could detect and free these blockages, thus healing the body.

What It's Good For • Therapeutic touch practitioners claim it can be used to ease a variety of ailments, including arthritis, chronic back pain, headaches, constipation, and colic in babies. Practitioners also report it can help wounds and broken bones to heal faster and can reduce fevers. Therapeutic touch is frequently used to reduce stress and anxiety. It has been used in some hospitals, for example, to relax people before and after surgery and to alleviate pain.

Preparations/Techniques • Despite its name, therapeutic touch does not involve actual physical contact. Each session begins with the practitioner assuming a relaxed, meditative state. The practitioner then moves his or her hands in slow, rhythmic motions 2–6 in (5–15 cm) above the patient in an effort to detect blockages in the body's energy field that may be causing or contributing to illness. When perceiving a blockage, the practitioner 'unruffles' the field with a downward sweep of the hands. After this, the practitioner transfers energy to the patient via what is called non-contact touch. Sessions last about 20 minutes. Once you become proficient in the technique, you can practise it on yourself and on others.

Well-being • Therapeutic touch is most commonly used to relieve pain and other symptoms of illness, but some practitioners also use the technique to help prevent the body from becoming ill in the first place.

What the Critics Say
Although conceding that the technique may comfort some patients, critics of therapeutic touch say that its healing value has not been demonstrated in well-designed, controlled scientific studies.

Target Ailments

- Arthritis
- Back Problems
- Bronchitis
- Bursitis
- Cancer
- Circulatory Problems
- Constipation
- Endometriosis
- Headache
- Heart Problems
- High Blood Pressure
- Immune Problems
- Menopause Problems
- Menstrual Problems
- Pain, Chronic
- Stress

FOR MORE INFO
Contact the following organizations to learn more about therapeutic touch:

Sacred Space Foundation
017687 79000

CONTINUED

Body Work CONTINUED

Target Ailments

■ Back Problems

■ Headache

■ Multiple Sclerosis

■ Pain, Chronic

■ TMJ Syndrome

Trager Psychophysical Integration (Trager Approach)

This type of body work was first developed in the 1920s by a young Miami boxer named Milton Trager, who was told by relatives and friends that he had an uncanny knack for massaging away their aches and pains. He eventually gave up boxing to become a physical therapist and later a doctor, and over the next seven decades treated thousands of patients with his unique and gentle form of massage. In the 1970s Trager began teaching his technique to others, who now offer it in the United States and other countries to people seeking relief from chronic pain and other ailments.

What It's Good For • The Trager approach is used in the treatment of all kinds of chronic pain, including back pain, headaches, muscle spasms and TMJ syndrome. A few small studies have shown it to be beneficial for some people with severe neuromuscular problems produced by injury or with such diseases as multiple sclerosis or muscular dystrophy.

Preparations/Techniques • Sessions last 60 to 90 minutes. The patient lies or sits on a table while the practitioner applies gentle touch and rhythmic rocking and shaking movements to the body to relax and loosen joints and muscles. Practitioners work in a meditative state called hook-up, which enables them to better sense minute responses of the patient's body. Patients are also taught a series of exercises to practise at home. Called mentastics, they are intended to help identify and correct chronic tension patterns that affect posture and movement.

Well-being • Trager practitioners believe that this form of movement re-education brings people into a relaxed and physically graceful state that enhances wellness and helps make the body more resistant to injury and illness.

What the Critics Say

Because large, controlled studies involving the Trager approach to body work have never been conducted, its ability to help people suffering from chronic pain or other ailments cannot be stated with any degree of certainty. ■

FOR MORE INFO

Contact the following organization to learn more about the Trager approach:

The Trager Institute
21 Locust Avenue
Mill Valley, CA 94941-2806
USA
e-mail: TragerD@aol.com

Chinese Medicine

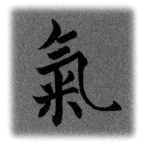

C hinese medicine is an ancient system of healthcare that uses a variety of techniques—including acupuncture (pages 22-23), acupressure (pages 6-7), herbal therapy (pages 56-59), qigong (pages 134-135) and massage (pages 92-94)—to treat disorders by restoring the balance of vital energies in the body.

Unlike Western medicine, which tends to focus on specific parts of the body immediately affected by disease or injury, Chinese medicine takes a more global, holistic approach to healthcare, fashioning remedies to treat the entire body rather than just its component parts. Practitioners of Chinese medicine think of the human body not as a bundle of cells, bones, and tissues but rather as a complex system of interrelated processes—an ecosystem unto itself, constantly influenced by the push and pull of opposing forces within it. These doctors regard the human being as both a part of nature and a separate entity, complete and self-contained. It is, they believe, a microcosm of the grand cosmic order, moved by the same rhythms and cycles that shape the natural world. At the core of Chinese medicine is the belief that disease is the result of disturbances in the flow of a bodily energy called chi or qi (pronounced 'chee') or a lack of balance in the complementary states of yin (characterized by darkness and quiet) and yang (characterized by light and activity).

Chi and the Dynamics of Yin and Yang

Defined in early Chinese writings as 'basic stuff', chi is thought to be the force that animates life and enlivens all activity. Powerful yet invisible, chi cannot be isolated, measured, or quantified; it is known not through direct observation but through its observable effects. Just as blood courses through the vessels of the circulatory system, chi flows through the body primarily by way of invisible channels called meridians. Practitioners of Chinese medicine believe that maintaining the proper movement of chi through these meridians is essential to good health.

Well-being also requires preserving a delicate balance, or equilibrium, between the contrasting states of yin and yang. Translated literally, the Chinese character for *yin* depicts the shady side of the mountain, *yang* the sunny side; together they symbolize the dual nature of all things. According to Chinese theory, yin and yang co-exist harmoniously in the body. Polar opposites, they represent alternate phases in the natural cycle, contradicting and at the same time complementing one another. In a healthy body, the darkness and inactivity of yin are perfectly counterbalanced

Target Ailments

- Allergies
- Arthritis
- Asthma
- Bursitis
- Common Cold
- Constipation
- Depression
- Diarrhoea
- Earache
- Flu
- Haemorrhoids
- Headache
- High Blood Pressure
- Insomnia
- Menstrual Problems
- Nausea
- Pain, Chronic
- Sore Throat
- Stomach Ulcers
- Stress
- Vaginal Problems

CONTINUED

Chinese Medicine

by the lightness and activity of yang. Just as day melts into night and night into day, the body fluctuates cyclically between yin and yang. Any deviation from this orderly course causes a yin-yang disharmony, resulting in disease.

Origins

Rooted in the philosophies of Taoism, Buddhism and Confucianism, Chinese medicine has been practised in China for more than 2,500 years, although the underlying principles of herbal therapy and acupuncture are even older. According to legend, the philosophical and practical groundwork of Chinese herbal medicine was laid by Emperor Shen Nung, the 'Divine Farmer' who became fascinated with the apparent healing properties of certain plants. He spent years testing the efficacy of these herbs, and his observations led him to develop a theory involving nature's 'opposing principles'. In the centuries that followed, Chinese thinkers refined and elaborated on these principles, which came to be called yin and yang. The philosophy grew and flourished in China, and from there spread throughout much of eastern Asia. However, it remained relatively unknown in the West until just a few decades ago.

What It's Good For

Chinese medicine is used to treat a full spectrum of conditions. In recent years these methods have been subjected to increasingly rigorous study both in China and elsewhere in the world. Evidence indicates that, although some may not perform as claimed, a number of these remedies do seem to work. For example, acupuncture has been shown to be effective in the treatment of nausea, asthma and migraines. In other studies, researchers have found that the management of chronic pain and drug addiction is more successful when acupuncture is included in a comprehensive treatment plan.

Preparations/Techniques

Chinese medicine recognizes more than 6,000 healing substances, although only a few hundred are in practical use today. Following a sophisticated classification system, herbs are grouped according to four basic properties, or 'essences'— hot, cold, warm and cool. In general, practitioners choose plants for their ability to restore balance in individuals whose conditions are said to show signs of excessive heat or cold. For example, a hot herb such as cinnamon bark might be recommended for a condition described as cold; the cool herb chrysanthemum flower might be prescribed for a condition characterized as warm.

Herbs are further categorized according to their 'flavour'—pungent, sour, sweet, bitter or salty. A herb's taste indicates its action in the body, particularly on the

Chinese Medicine

movement and direction of chi. Each flavour is said to have a strong influence on a certain major organ system: pungent herbs are associated with the lungs, sour with the liver, sweet with the spleen or pancreas, bitter with the heart, salty with the kidneys. It is important to note that the Chinese notion of body organs is much broader than the Western. The Chinese term for *heart,* for instance, encompasses not only the physical organ itself but also the general order and clarity of the mind.

Because many Chinese herbs work best when taken with others, practitioners almost always prescribe herbs in combination, occasionally blending as many as 15 in a single preparation. Some plants are used to disperse chi that has become stagnant or misdirected. Others help summon scattered reserves of chi, while still others provide nourishment or rid the body of noxious substances.

Herbs are prepared in a variety of ways. Many are cooked and made into soup or tea. In some cases the raw plants are ground into a powder, then combined with honey or some other binding agent and pressed into a pill. A number of herbs are cooked and processed into a powder and are then either mixed with warm water and swallowed or taken as capsules. Some herbs are made into pastes that are applied to the skin, while others are extracted in alcohol and used as tinctures. Mixing herbs is an extremely tricky business. Certain Chinese herbs can be poisonous if consumed in large enough amounts, so you should always check with a qualified practitioner for the proper dosages.

Before prescribing any type of treatment, a practitioner performs an evaluation of the patient's overall physical and mental makeup, or 'individual conformation'. According to Chinese theory, a single symptom by itself is meaningless; it acquires significance only in terms of how it relates to a host of other signs. The evaluation consists of four basic techniques, or stages: looking, listening and smelling (in Chinese, these are expressed by the same word), asking and touching.

An experienced practitioner can gather a great deal of information by observing the patient's general appearance, posture, facial colour, and behaviour. For more detailed information, the doctor looks for more specific signs, such as the alertness of the eyes and the colour of the skin and nails. Crucial to the diagnosis is a careful evaluation of the patient's tongue, which is considered to be an excellent barometer of disharmonies in the body. To trained eyes, the shape, movement, colour, texture and moistness of the tongue—even its coating—speak volumes about the patient's condition. A red, dry tongue, for example, suggests the presence of heat; whilst a purple tongue may indicate stagnant chi. During their examinations, practitioners take pulse readings at three points on each wrist; each point is believed to reveal conditions in different parts of the body. They also look for clues in bodily secretions, the sound of the voice and any unusual odours that may be emanating from the patient's body.

CONTINUED

Chinese Medicine CONTINUED

Chinese Medicine and Well-being

Preventing disease and preserving the conditions of good health are among the fundamental aims of Chinese medicine. More than a system of after-the-fact healing techniques, it is a philosophy of life grounded on the assumption that illness is much easier to prevent than to cure. Besides providing treatment to overcome disease, practitioners strive to arm the body against conditions that bring about ill health. Historically, Chinese medical professionals have rejected the notion of quick cures, insisting that disease is caused by deep-rooted imbalances that must be treated continuously over time. (In ancient China, doctors were paid only if their patients stayed healthy.) Herbal therapy, in particular, is often prescribed to be used on a regular basis to correct small energy imbalances before they can erupt into major problems. Many Chinese herbs can be taken or eaten daily as a preventive measure in much the same way as vitamins or nutritional supplements.

What the Critics Say

Many of those raised in the tradition of Western medicine dismiss Chinese medicine as so much superstition and hocus-pocus—a vague, primitive, and quasi-religious set of beliefs founded not on the principles of hard science and logical reasoning but on irrational faith and mysticism. They refute claims that Chinese medicine is appropriate for all ailments, and they attribute any positive results to other causes or to simple good luck. Nonetheless, recent studies have shown that Chinese medical techniques can be effective. Acupuncture, in particular, has proved to be especially beneficial in chronic pain management, stroke rehabilitation, drug addiction and nausea relief. Inserting needles in the skin evidently releases endorphins and other chemicals that serve as the body's natural painkillers, although how acupuncture provides long-term pain management is unclear.

Barriers are gradually falling, and now certain medical practices of the East are starting to gain formal acceptance in cultures of the West. In one sign of this newfound recognition, the World Health Organization of the United Nations lists about 50 diseases for which it considers acupuncture an appropriate treatment. ∎

FOR MORE INFO

Following is a list of organizations you can contact to learn more about Chinese medicine:

British Acupuncture Council
63 Jeddo Road
London W12 9HQ
020 8735 0400
fax: 020 08735 0404

British Medical Acupuncture Society
01925 730 727
Members are doctors.

Foundation for Traditional Chinese Medicine
122a Acomb Road
York YO24 4EY
01904 781 630

Register of Chinese Herbal Medicine
30 Albion Yard
London E1 1BY

Institute for Complementary Medicine
PO Box 194
London SE16 1QZ
fax: 020 7237 5175

Chiropractic

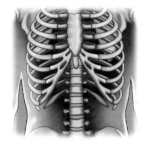

C hiropractic is based on the concept that the human body has an innate self-healing ability and seeks homoeostasis, or balance. According to general chiropractic theory, the nervous system plays an important role in maintaining homoeostasis—and hence health. But 'subluxations' (misalignments of bones within joints) or 'fixations' (abnormalities of motion) are said to interfere with the flow of nervous impulses and diminish the body's ability to stay healthy. Through manipulation of the bones and their associated muscles and joints, particularly the spine, chiropractors work to correct these misalignments, thereby improving the function of the neuromusculoskeletal system and restoring homoeostasis. The term chiropractic is derived from the Greek words 'cheir' (hand) and 'practikos' (done by).

Today, chiropractors are divided into two major camps. On one side are the straights—traditional chiropractors who adhere to the philosophy that subluxations are at the root of disease and that manipulation is the best treatment. On the other side are the mixers, so named because their approach represents a mix of traditional and progressive techniques.

Although chiropractic is often considered alternative medicine, it is gaining wider acceptance, in part because of recent clinical studies showing these methods to be effective in treating problems such as acute lower back pain and headache.

Target Ailments

- Arthritis
- Asthma
- Back Problems
- Bursitis
- Carpal Tunnel Syndrome
- Chronic Fatigue Syndrome
- Earache
- Headache
- High Blood Pressure
- Menstrual Problems
- Muscle Cramps
- Neuralgia
- Pain, Chronic
- Premenstrual Syndrome
- Sprains and Strains
- Tendinitis
- TMJ Syndrome

Origins

Chiropractic originated in 1895, when Daniel David Palmer, a magnetic healer who practised laying on of hands in Davenport, Iowa, cured a janitor's deafness by pushing on a malpositioned vertebra in the man's back. To Palmer, this was proof that misalignments in the spine could impair health and that realigning the spine enhanced health by restoring the flow of nerve impulses throughout the body.

Two years later Palmer founded the first chiropractic school, and it was here, under the management of his son, that the schism currently dividing the profession began to form. Dissatisfied with the Palmers' teachings—particularly their claims about the role of subluxations in disease—a faculty member named John Howard broke away to start his own chiropractic college (now the National College of Chiropractic). Using many of Palmer's theories, Howard set about developing a programme that was more firmly grounded in rational thought and solid scientific evidence. Within less than a decade, a number of other chiropractic schools had emerged. Those practitioners who allied themselves with the Palmers became known

CONTINUED

Chiropractic CONTINUED

as the straights; whilst those who departed from the original concept were dubbed the mixers.

The straight-mixer split began a debate within the chiropractic community over the scope of its techniques and the profession's relationship with conventional medicine. While the straights concentrate almost exclusively on manipulation, the mixers employ manipulation along with a broad range of other therapeutic methods, including massage, physical therapy and nutritional therapy.

What It's Good For

Straight chiropractors believe that chiropractic manipulation can provide relief from every type of ailment, from asthma to impotence. The mixers, on the other hand, maintain that chiropractic is appropriate only for certain conditions and is particularly effective in the treatment of acute lower back pain, musculoskeletal problems, headache and neck pain.

- **Back pain:** Studies show that spinal manipulation can relieve acute lower back pain, the most common reason that people make their first visit to a chiropractor.
- **Neck pain:** Chiropractic adjustment can often help correct painful misalignments in the neck, including those caused by whiplash injury.
- **Headache:** Spinal manipulation has been shown to decrease the frequency and intensity of migraine and tension headaches.
- **Other conditions:** Scientific studies and anecdotal evidence suggest that chiropractic can be beneficial in the treatment of otitis media, digestive problems, dysmenorrhoea, hypertension, disc problems, scoliosis, sprains and some sports injuries, frozen shoulder, tennis elbow, carpal tunnel syndrome, abnormal jaw function, respiratory problems, enuresis and arthritis in the wrist, hand or hip.

Visiting a Professional

Your first visit to a chiropractor usually begins with a general evaluation and case history. While noting your posture and gait, the practitioner will ask you about the problem and how it began, and about your medical history and lifestyle.

For the actual examination, you will be asked to wear a hospital gown. The chiropractor will palpate, or feel, your vertebrae to detect misplacement of bones or muscle weakness, and may perform a reflex test to check nerve function. You will then be instructed to bend forward, backward and sideways while the chiropractor palpates your vertebrae and joints to determine their range of motion. The doctor may also take X-rays in order to discover any joint problems that could be worsened by manipulation.

Chiropractic

Next, the doctor will make a diagnosis and determine a treatment plan, which may begin right away or on your second visit. In chiropractic treatment the practitioner adjusts your joints using a small controlled thrust that moves the joint slightly beyond its restricted range of motion; before making the adjustment, however, the doctor may massage the area around the joint in order to loosen tight muscles and ligaments.

If the chiropractor is adjusting your spine, you will need to lie on a padded table on your stomach or side. For an adjustment of your neck, you will be asked to sit upright. (While adjustments are being made, you may hear the joints crack just as your knuckles do when they crack.) The treatments are painless, and many patients feel improvement within nine to 12 sessions.

Well-being

Unless you have a musculoskeletal problem, chiropractic may not fit into your long-term health plan. Some chiropractors insist that manipulation should be used to treat only specific problems, and that manipulating a healthy spine or joint accomplishes nothing. Others, however, argue that periodic chiropractic adjustments should be part of a preventive health maintenance programme.

What the Critics Say

- Some medical doctors maintain that misaligned vertebrae—the chiropractor's clue to health problems—are common, often harmless, and do not require treatment.
- Critics charge that frequent visits to a chiropractor are useless, whether as a preventive measure or to treat a specific condition such as back pain—which, they say, usually clears up on its own.
- Those critical of chiropractic often point out that quadriplegics can have healthy internal organs despite their extensive nerve damage. This fact, they maintain, disproves the assertion that a sound nervous system is the key to overall health.
- A number of critics argue that chiropractors should restrict their practice to treating back pain, since there is insufficient evidence to show that manipulation provides relief from any other condition.

FOR MORE INFO
Following is a list of organizations you can contact to learn more about chiropractic medicine:

General Chiropractic Council
344–354 Gray's Inn Road
3rd floor, North Wing
London WC1X 8BP
020 7713 5155
fax: 020 7713 5844

Chiropractic Patients' Association
8 Centre One
Lysander Way
Old Sarum
Salisbury SP4 6BU
01722 415 027
fax: 01722 415 028
email: c.p.a.@dial.pipex.com

Institute for Complementary Medicine
PO Box 194
London SE16 1QZ
fax: 020 7237 5175

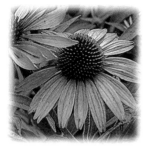

Target Ailments

- Athletic Injuries
- Back Problems
- Chronic Fatigue Syndrome
- Depression
- Headache
- Immune Problems
- Insomnia
- Pain, Chronic
- Premenstrual Syndrome
- Stress

Flower Remedies

F lower remedies, also called flower essences, are specially prepared liquid concentrates made by soaking flowers in pure spring water. The concentrates are diluted and sipped to treat various emotional and physical disorders. The fundamental theory behind flower-essence therapy is that physical ailments and disease, as well as psychological problems, arise from emotional disturbances; diagnosis and treatment thus involve an evaluation of personality, state of mind and emotional makeup.

Like homoeopathic remedies (pages 77-79), flower essences are diluted to such a degree that they do not work on a biochemical level. Practitioners say they contain specific aspects of the plants' energy, which affect the energy field of the person taking them. In this way, the flower remedies are believed to help people work with and integrate their emotions; a typical treatment might, for example, aim to develop in a fearful person the courage to face his or her fear.

Origins

Although healing with flowers goes back to ancient times, the specific use of flower concentrates to treat emotions and attitudes was developed in the 1930s by the English bacteriologist and homoeopathic doctor Edward Bach. After careful observation of his patients, Bach concluded not only that links existed between certain personality traits and certain illnesses but also that people with similar personalities reacted to their illnesses similarly. He searched for natural agents that would deal with the emotional precursors to disease and eventually discovered the flower essences, whose specific qualities he determined through intuition and experimentation on himself.

Today, many companies produce versions of flower essences. Among the major, well-established lines are the original 38 English essences of Dr Bach, available from several different sources; North American flower essences, a group of over 100 remedies sometimes called California remedies; and a series of Rose essences, some of which are designated as addressing specific functions of the body.

What It's Good For

Proponents say flower remedies are helpful for numerous physical ailments and emotional states. Each of Bach's original 38 remedies corresponds to a negative mood or state of mind. The 38 are divided into seven groups of emotions: fear, uncertainty, insufficient interest in present circumstances, loneliness, oversensitivity to influences and ideas, despondency and despair, and overconcern for the welfare of

Flower Remedies

others. Within each of the seven groups are subcategories of the emotion, each with a specific remedy. For example, subcategories under fear include terror, fear of an unknown cause and fear for other people.

The group of English remedies includes a combination formula of five of the 38 essences that is said to be beneficial for a variety of problems, such as physical injury, shock, pain, or severe emotional upset. Among the brand names for this combination are Rescue Remedy, Five Flower Formula and Calming Essence.

Preparations/Techniques

The remedies, usually obtained in liquid concentrate form (called the stock) and preserved in alcohol or vinegar, may be bought at health food shops and some chemists, by mail order or through a practitioner. Preparation of the essences is a complex process that takes into account a variety of factors, including the plants' environment and the climatic conditions at the time of collection and concentration.

You can match your own emotions and state of mind with those listed in the chart on pages 54-55 to choose one or more remedies (up to six at a time) for yourself or your children. To administer, place 2 to 4 drops of the stock under your tongue four times daily or place several drops in a large glass of water and sip a few times a day. Flower essences may also be used topically or added to baths.

Visiting a Professional

If you are unfamiliar with these remedies, it may be helpful to seek out a practitioner at first. The practitioner is likely to choose your remedies by observing you and asking you questions, and possibly by evaluating the results of certain physical tests.

What the Critics Say

Critics point out that claims of effectiveness are based on intuition rather than science and therefore are unsubstantiated. Some say any reported positive effects are due to the placebo effect; however, proponents point to benefits experienced by animals and children, who presumably would not be susceptible to the placebo effect. Proponents also claim there is no evidence of side effects, ill effects following a wrong diagnosis, or harmful interactions with any other medicines. ■

CAUTION

Some practitioners say that the essences may bring unresolved emotional issues to the surface for consideration, which may be psychologically unsettling, yet beneficial in the long run.

People who are sensitive to the alcohol in some remedies can dilute the remedy or use a few drops on the wrist or lips rather than ingesting.

FOR MORE INFO

Contact the following organization to learn more about flower essences:

Doctor Edward Bach Centre
Mount Vernon
Bakers Lane
Sotwell
Wallingford
Oxfordshire OX10 0PZ
01491 834 678

CONTINUED

39 Essential Flower Remedies

This chart lists the 38 Bach essences plus the combination formula Rescue Remedy. Each entry describes—in language typically used by practitioners—the mental and emotional states for which that remedy is said to be beneficial. Up to six Bach remedies may be taken at a time. The illustrations show four common herbs from which additional essences—beyond Bach's originals—have been developed.

Agrimony
Proclivity to conceal worry and deny pain, restlessness, distressed by arguments and confrontation.

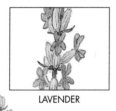

LAVENDER

Aspen
Unexplained anxiety, apprehension, fears of unknown origin, tending to have nightmares.

Beech
Intolerant, critical, dissatisfied, negative, unwilling to make allowances.

Centaury
Weak-willed, submissive, easily influenced or imposed upon, difficulty saying no.

Cerato
Distrust of self and own ability, overdependent on the advice of others.

Cherry Plum
Desperation, fear of emotional breakdown, uncontrolled and irrational thoughts.

Chestnut Bud
Failure to learn from experience, lack of observation, repeating mistakes.

Chicory
Possessiveness, self-love, self-pity, controlling, demanding, attention-seeking.

Clematis
Indifference, daydreaming, inattention, absorbed in own thoughts, impractical.

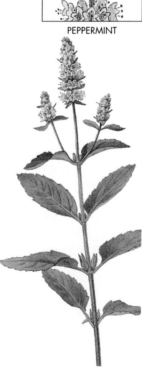

PEPPERMINT

Crab Apple
Self-disgust, shame, feeling of uncleanness.

Elm
Occasional feelings of inadequacy, being overwhelmed by responsibility.

Gentian
Doubt, depression, discouragement after setback, scepticism, negativity.

Gorse
Hopelessness, despair, resignation, loss of will, pessimism, defeatism.

Heather
Self-centred, talking incessantly about oneself, obsessed with own problems.

Holly
Hatred, envy, jealousy, suspicion, strong negativity, feeling cut off from love.

Honeysuckle
Nostalgia, homesickness, living in the past, regretful, loss of interest in the present.

Hornbeam
Fatigue, feeling of

Flower Remedies

being burdened, temporary mental and physical exhaustion, procrastination.

Impatiens
Impatience, irritability, intolerance, impulsivity, nervous tension, over-exertion.

Larch
Lack of confidence, despondency, self-censorship, feelings of inferiority.

Mimulus
Fear or anxiety of known things, timidity, shyness, nervousness.

Mustard
Deep depression of unknown cause, sadness that comes and goes unexpectedly.

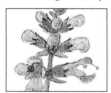

SAGE

Oak
Plodding, uncomplaining, inflexible, over-achieving, obstinate.

Olive
Complete exhaustion, depletion after illness or long-term stress.

Pine
Self-reproach, guilt, self-blame, inability to accept self, apologetic.

Red Chestnut
Excessive fear or anxiety for loved ones, anticipation of trouble.

Rock Rose
Sudden alarm, terror, panic, hysteria, nightmares, feelings of horror.

Rock Water
Self-repression, self-denial, self-martyrdom, perfectionism, obsessiveness.

Scleranthus
Uncertainty, indecision, hesitancy, confusion, wavering, lack of mental clarity.

Star-of-Bethlehem
Grief, distress, past or

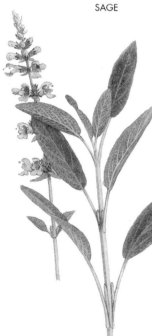

> ### ■ RESCUE REMEDY
> **Star-of-Bethlehem, Rock Rose, Impatiens, Cherry Plum, Clematis**
> Trauma, terror, panic, stress, desperation, disorientation.

present trauma such as that sustained from bad news, accident, or fright.

Sweet Chestnut
Extreme mental anguish, utter dejection, hopelessness, despair.

Vervain
Over-enthusiastic, tendency to impose will, argumentative, fanatical, overbearing.

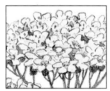

YARROW

Vine
Dominating others, tyrannical, ambitious, arrogant, inflexible, ruthless.

Walnut
Difficulty in adjusting to transition or change, including relocation, a new job, divorce, menopause or puberty.

Water Violet
Pride, aloofness, self-reliance, non-interfering, enjoys being alone.

White Chestnut
Persistent unwanted thoughts, internal arguments, worry, preoccupation.

Wild Oat
Dissatisfaction due to uncertainty regarding career, lack of direction or commitment.

Wild Rose
Resignation, apathy, surrender, failure to make effort, lack of hope.

Willow
Resentment, bitterness, grumbling, self-pity, blaming others, dissatisfaction, victim role.

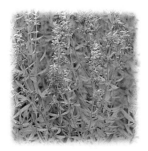

*H*erbal Therapies

Target Ailments

Herbs are used for ailments affecting all body systems.

- Cardiovascular System
- Digestive System
- Immune System
- Musculoskeletal System
- Nervous System
- Reproductive System
- Respiratory System
- Skin
- Urinary System

Herbal medicines are prepared from a wide variety of plant materials—frequently the leaves, stems, roots and bark, but also the flowers, fruits, twigs, seeds and exudates (material that oozes out, such as sap). They generally contain several biologically active ingredients and are used primarily for treating chronic or mild conditions, although on occasion they are employed as complementary or supportive therapy for acute and severe diseases.

Across the spectrum of alternative medicine, the use of herbs is varied: Western herbology, Chinese medicine and Ayurvedic medicine differ in the way practitioners diagnose diseases and prescribe herbal remedies. Naturopaths may use herbs from any of these systems.

Western Herbs

Medicinal plants in the group known as Western herbs bear English as well as Latin names and are categorized in several ways. Normalizers, or tonics, have a gentle, healing effect on the body. Another type, called effectors, have powerful actions and are used to treat illnesses. Herbs are also frequently grouped into more than 20 categories according to how they affect the body. Some of these categories are familiar—anti-inflammatories, diuretics, laxatives. Other, less well known classes include diaphoretics (herbs that promote perspiration and therefore the elimination of waste products through the skin) and nervines (herbs that act to strengthen the nervous system).

In many cases, herbs are also grouped according to the body systems they affect. The cardiovascular system, for example, responds well to herbs that strengthen blood vessels; these herbs include ginkgo, buckwheat and linden. The digestive system, on the other hand, benefits from the relaxing effects of chamomile. Individual herbs can act on a body system in different ways. For instance, the sedative valerian, the cardiotonic herb hawthorn and the herb St John's wort, which has an antidepressant effect, invoke distinct responses from the nervous system.

Traditional Chinese Herbs

Another group of herbs, used by practitioners of Chinese medicine, are part of a larger system of healing that attempts to help the body correct energy imbalances *(see Chinese Medicine, pages 45-48)*. Chinese herbs are classified according to certain active characteristics (such as heating, cooling, moisturizing or drying) and are prescribed according to how they influence the various organ systems. Practitioners of Chinese medicine also recognize five herb 'tastes'—sweet, sour,

Herbal Therapies

salty, pungent and bitter—each of which is associated with a particular physiological action. Chinese herbal prescriptions usually contain several herbs, perhaps as many as a dozen. These combinations are chosen not only for their effect on specific diseases but also for their ability to balance potential side effects and direct the therapy to a certain area of the body.

Origins

People have used plants for medicine since before recorded history, and all known cultures have long histories of folk medicine that include the use of herbs. Physical evidence of the existence of herbal remedies was found in the burial site of a Neanderthal man who lived more than 60,000 years ago.

Early observations of the characteristics of herbs and the way certain plants affected animals and humans were amassed in collections called pharmacopoeias or materia medicas. Many traditional herbalists believed that a healing energy inherent in the plants, and not just the chemical constituents alone, accounted for the beneficial effects of herbal remedies—a theory that is being explored by some contemporary practitioners.

Ancient cultures such as those of Greece and Rome developed well-defined herbal pharmacopoeias, and some herbal knowledge came to Europe from the Middle East during the Crusades. In the US and Britain, herbs were used for many years to prevent various ailments and treat minor emergencies. In fact, doctors relied on herbal preparations as primary medicines through the 1930s.

During the latter part of the 20th century, the use of plant remedies declined with advancements in medical technology and developments in the production of new pharmaceuticals. A 1992 report on alternative medicine prepared for the US National Institutes of Health expressed concern that our knowledge of herbs—as medicinal plants and as unique species—may soon be lost. Recently, however, interest in herbal therapy has increased dramatically, partly in response to the growing perception that medicinal drugs are expensive, may cause side effects or allergic reactions and are not capable of curing every disease.

What It's Good For

Herbal therapy offers remedies for virtually every ailment affecting all body systems. For a list of specific herbs and some of their medicinal uses, see The 50 Most Effective Herbs on pages 60-76.

Preparations/Techniques

Herbs are available in various forms at health food shops and chemists, and many can be ordered by mail. Although Chinese herbs can sometimes be bought at

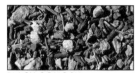

BLACK COHOSH

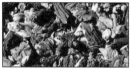

DANDELION

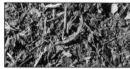

NETTLE

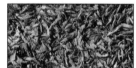

RED CLOVER

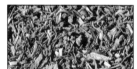

VALERIAN

Dried Herbs • *The leaves and other parts of medicinal plants, including those shown above, are sold in many forms.*

CONTINUED

Herbal Therapies CONTINUED

Asian food stores, these products are more likely to be dispensed by practitioners, who are familiar with the combination formulas. Many practitioners of Chinese medicine also dispense Western herbs.

Herbal remedies can be prepared at home in a variety of different ways, using either fresh or dried ingredients. Herbal teas, or infusions, can be steeped to varying strengths. Roots, bark or other plant parts can be simmered into strong solutions called decoctions. Honey or sugar can be added to infusions and decoctions to make syrups. You can also purchase many herbal remedies over the counter in the form of pills, capsules or powders, as well as in more concentrated liquid forms called extracts and tinctures. Certain herbs can be applied topically as creams or ointments, soaked into cloths and used as compresses, or applied directly to the skin as poultices.

Visiting a Professional

Because some herbs can be toxic or carcinogenic, all medicinal plants should be used only under the guidance of a practitioner who is familiar with herbal medicine. The major professional herbalists include naturopaths specializing in botanical medicine, acupuncturists trained in Chinese herbal medicine, Ayurvedic doctors and trained medical or clinical herbalists.

Practitioners select a plant or formula that is appropriate for the patient rather than for just the complaint alone. Typically, the herbalist will take your personal and family history and may either perform a physical examination or request the results of a recent exam. He or she may evaluate any personal, social or lifestyle factors that affect your health, then make recommendations regarding diet, exercise or other lifestyle modifications. The practitioner will then suggest one or more remedies deemed appropriate for your condition. The exact form and dosage will depend on the strength of the herb, the effects desired, your age and your constitution. In the case of Chinese medicine, the choice of herbs is based on a diagnostic system that evaluates specific individual characteristics, including the pulse rate and the appearance of the tongue *(see Chinese Medicine, pages 45-48)*.

Well-being

Herbs can be of great value when used in a programme of self-care and preventive medicine. But because they vary in strength from gentle remedies that can be eaten like food to potential lethal poisons, medicinal plants should always be used under the supervision of a professional. A practitioner can advise which of the milder 'tonic' herbs, such as dandelion and nettle, are safe and appropriate for your particular condition. A number of culinary herbs may also be used in a preventive health programme.

Herbal Therapies

What the Critics Say

Those suspicious of herbal therapy often point to the widespread availability of what they consider inaccurate or deceptive information about herbs. Although herbs cannot legally be labelled as to their efficacy in fighting diseases, literature—some of it carrying extreme claims of therapeutic effectiveness—may be sold alongside herbs on store shelves. Sometimes dangerous herbs are recommended, and in other cases herbs are said to be imbued with magical or mystical properties. Such claims draw fire from critics either because they are unscientific or because they leave the erroneous impression that potentially dangerous plants are harmless.

Herbal therapy also is criticized because medicinal plants have not been tested for efficacy according to rigid pharmaceutical standards. However, these tests are very expensive. Because herbs are natural products and cannot be patented, any company paying for such testing would likely never recover its losses. Furthermore, there's continuing debate over whether such testing should be performed on the entire herb or only on its active ingredients. Some remedies depend on the actions of several components (or several herbs) working together. Another problem is that sometimes a herb's active ingredients are not actually known.

Proponents of herbal therapy point out that the pharmaceutical industry grew out of herbal treatment and that plant extracts are still used to make drugs. For example, digitalis, used to treat heart disease, comes from the foxglove, and morphine comes from the opium poppy. About 25 per cent of today's prescription drugs are at least partially derived from plants. ∎

OF SPECIAL INTEREST

Using Herbs Safely

Purchasing herbs is generally safer than harvesting your own plants. Many herbalists also advise against collecting your own herbs from the wild. Plants have natural variations that can be misleading, and the consequences of a mistake can be severe. A number of people have died from ingesting toxic wild plants believed to be benign substances. Because all forms of herbs lose potency over time, you should look for a source that provides the freshest possible product.

If you consistently develop nausea, diarrhoea or headache within two hours of taking a herb, discontinue its use immediately. Call your practitioner if the symptoms are prolonged. Women who are pregnant or breastfeeding are advised not to take medicinal amounts of herbs without first consulting a doctor.

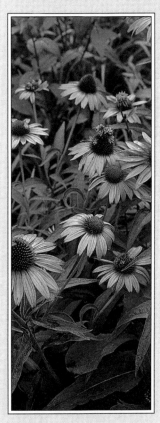

Echinacea

Aloe
Aloe barbadensis

The translucent gel obtained from the inner leaves of this tropical herb works externally to relieve minor burns, skin irritations, and infections; taken internally, it provides relief from stomach disorders. Among its ingredients are several that reduce inflammation. Aloe gel is also used as a beauty aid and moisturizer because it contains polysaccharides, which act as emollients.

■ TARGET AILMENTS
Take internally for digestive disorders, gastritis, stomach ulcers.
Apply externally for minor burns, infected wounds, insect bites, irritated skin or eyes, bruises, chickenpox, sunburn, acne.

PREPARATIONS
Over the counter: Aloe is available as powder, fluidextract, powdered capsules or bottled gel.
At home:
Eyewash: Dissolve ½ tsp powdered aloe gel in 8 fl oz (235 ml) water. Add 1 tsp boric acid to accelerate the healing process. Pour through a coffee filter before applying to the eyes.
Bath: Add 8–16 fl oz (235–475 ml) gel to a warm bath to relieve sunburn or skin lesions.
Combinations: Use aloe gel externally with wheat-germ oil and safflower flower to reduce bruising.

SIDE EFFECTS
Not serious: The use of aloe may result in allergic dermatitis, intestinal cramps or diarrhoea. Try a lower dosage or stop using the product.

SPECIAL INFORMATION
❧ If you are pregnant or have a gastrointestinal illness, consult a herbalist or doctor before taking aloe internally.

Astragalus
Astragalus membranaceus

The perennial plant astragalus, or milk-vetch root, has sprawling stems and pale yellow blooms. Western herbalists believe that substances known as polysaccharides in this herb stimulate the immune system and generally strengthen the body, promoting tissue regeneration, speeding metabolism and increasing energy. The herb is also used in traditional Chinese medicine.

■ TARGET AILMENTS
Take internally for general weakness & fatigue, appetite loss, spontaneous perspiration, diarrhoea, blood abnormalities, chronic colds and flu, AIDS, cancer. (Take with conventional medical treatment.)

PREPARATIONS
Over the counter: Astragalus is available as prepared tea, fluidextract, capsules and dried root.
At home:
Chinese: Combine 1 part honey, 4 parts dried root, and a small amount of water in a wok or frying pan. Allow mixture to simmer until the water evaporates and the herbs are slightly brown.
Combinations: For spontaneous perspiration, astragalus is mixed with Asian ginseng. As an immune system stimulant, the herb is combined with siler (*Ledebouriella divaricata*). Blood abnormalities are treated with a mix of astragalus and dong quai. Herbalists combine astragalus and atractylodes (white) for diarrhoea.
Western: Boil 1 oz (30 g) astragalus root in 8 fl oz (235 ml) water for 15 to 20 minutes to make a tea.

SIDE EFFECTS
None expected.

SPECIAL INFORMATION
❧ Pregnant women should check with their doctors before using astragalus.

Black Cohosh
Cimicifuga racemosa

The knotty black rhizome and root of black cohosh contain substances that act like the female hormone oestrogen. It is prescribed for several menstrual and menopausal conditions. The herb also acts as a sedative and is believed to promote urination, dry up discharges of fluid, aid in expelling mucus from the lungs and relieve coughing spasms.

■ **TARGET AILMENTS**
Take internally for menstrual discomfort, menopause, PMS, headache, bleeding gums, coughs.
Apply externally for sciatica, neuralgia, muscle spasms, rheumatism.

PREPARATIONS
Over the counter: Black cohosh is available as tincture, syrup, capsules, fluid extract, and also as dried root and rhizome.
At home:
Decoction: Boil ½ tsp powdered rootstock per 8 fl oz (235 ml) water for 30 minutes and let cool. Add lemon and honey. Take as much as this per day, 2 tbsp at a time.

SIDE EFFECTS
Not serious: Prolonged use may irritate the uterus.
Serious: Overdoses or prolonged use can cause dizziness, diarrhoea, nausea, vomiting, abdominal pain, headaches, joint pains and lowered heart rate. It can contribute to abnormal blood clotting, liver problems and breast tumours. If any symptoms develop, stop using black cohosh and call your doctor immediately.

SPECIAL INFORMATION
WARNING: Because it can cause serious side effects, use black cohosh only under medical supervision. Do not use if you have heart problems.
ఌ Do not use if you are pregnant or if you have been told not to take contraceptive pills.

Burdock
Arctium lappa

Herbalists have long prescribed burdock root for a wide range of illnesses. Today, some use it to treat urinary tract infections, arthritis, external wounds and skin ulcers. This herb works best in conjunction with conventional medical treatment. Burdock got its name from its tenacious burrs and from 'dock', the Old English word for plant.

■ **TARGET AILMENTS**
Take internally for fungal and bacterial infections; skin disorders, such as eczema and psoriasis, which cause dry, scaly skin; urinary tract infections; rheumatism; arthritis.
Apply externally for wounds and skin conditions.

PREPARATIONS
Over the counter: Burdock is available as dried powder, slices of root and tincture.
At home:
Decoction: Add 1 tsp burdock root to 24 fl oz (0.7 litre) water; boil for 30 minutes. Drink up to this amount a day to treat genital and urinary tract irritations.
Compress: Soak a clean cloth in burdock tea and place it on the skin to speed healing of wounds and skin ulcers.
Combinations: Burdock, mixed with yellow dock, red clover or cleavers, can be taken orally for skin disorders. Consult a herbalist for more information.

SPECIAL INFORMATION
WARNING: Because it stimulates the uterus, do not use if pregnant.
ఌ Do not give burdock to children younger than two years of age. Older children and people over 65 should start with lower-strength doses, increasing them if needed.
ఌ Doses higher than recommended may cause stomach discomfort.

Calendula
Calendula officinalis

The therapeutic use of calendula, whose medically active parts are its flowers, originated in ancient Egypt. One variety is the common marigold. A natural antiseptic and anti-inflammatory agent, calendula is one of the best herbs for treating wounds, skin abrasions, and infections. Taken internally, it also alleviates indigestion as well as other gastrointestinal disorders. Calendula's healing power appears to come from components known as terpenes. One of these is recognized as a sedative and for its healing effect on ulcers.

■ **TARGET AILMENTS**
Take internally for indigestion, gastric and duodenal ulcers, gallbladder problems, irregular or painful menstruation.
Apply externally for cuts, wounds, sores and burns; skin rashes from measles, chickenpox and other eruptive skin diseases; nappy rash; athlete's foot and other fungal infections.

PREPARATIONS
Over the counter: Available as lotion, ointment, oil, tincture and fresh or dried leaves and florets.
At home:
Rub lotions, ointments and oils on injuries, rashes and infections.
Poultice: Mash up the leaves, then apply directly to minor burns or scalds.
Tea: Steep 1 oz (30 g) dried herb in 16 fl. oz (435 ml) boiling water. For acute internal symptoms, drink two to four times a day until symptoms lessen.
Combinations: A mixture of goldenseal, calendula, and myrrh makes an antiseptic lotion.

SPECIAL INFORMATION
ఌ Calendula flowers can be made into an oil for external use and to ease earaches and other infections.

CONTINUED

The 50 Most Effective Herbs

Catnip
Nepeta cataria

Herbalists have used the flowers and leaves of catnip, an aromatic member of the mint family, for more than 2,000 years. Today it is prescribed for easing digestion, calming nerves and relieving muscle spasms, including menstrual cramps. Cats are strongly attracted to catnip and may become intoxicated by eating it, but the herb has no such effect on humans.

■ TARGET AILMENTS
Take internally for indigestion, gas, tension, difficulty in sleeping, colds, flu, bronchial congestion, fever, colic in infants, menstrual cramps.
Apply externally for cuts and scrapes.

PREPARATIONS
Over the counter: Catnip is available in dried bulk flowers and leaves, tincture and tea bags.
At home: To treat minor cuts and scrapes, press crushed catnip leaves into them before washing and bandaging them.

Tea: Pour 8 fl oz (235 ml) boiling water on to 2 tsp dried leaves and steep for 10 to 15 minutes. Drink three times a day.
Combinations: Mix with boneset, elder, yarrow or cayenne for colds.

SIDE EFFECTS
Not serious: Catnip can produce an upset stomach. If this occurs, discontinue use and call your doctor.

SPECIAL INFORMATION
- Avoid catnip during pregnancy.
- Infants with colic can be given weak, cool infusions. For older children and people over 65, start treatment with weak preparations and increase the strength as necessary.

Cayenne
Capsicum annuum var. annuum

Regarded by herbalists as a powerful tonic, cayenne stimulates the heart and promotes blood circulation, improves digestion and boosts energy. Like other species of hot pepper, such as tabasco, cayenne contains the natural stimulant known as capsaicin. Widely grown in Central and South America in pre-Columbian times, cayenne was carried to Spain and Europe after the early voyages of discovery.

■ TARGET AILMENTS
Take internally for poor circulation, indigestion, gas, physical or mental exhaustion and lowered vitality, particularly in the elderly.
Apply externally for pain, including that of arthritis and diabetes, strains, sore muscles and joints, the need to stimulate blood flow or to stop external bleeding.

PREPARATIONS
Over the counter: Available as powder, capsules, tincture or oil.
At home:
Rub the oil on sprains, swelling, sore muscles, and joints to ease pain.
Infusion: Pour 8 fl oz (235 ml) boiling water on to ½–1 tsp cayenne powder and steep for 10 minutes. Mix 1 tbsp of the infusion with hot water and drink as needed.
Gargle: Combine cayenne with myrrh to treat laryngitis and to use as an antiseptic wash.

SIDE EFFECTS
Not serious: In large doses, cayenne can produce vomiting, stomach pain and a type of intoxication. Do not exceed prescribed dosages.

SPECIAL INFORMATION
- Hot and spicy as a tea or tincture, cayenne can cause mild nausea at first. It's best to start with a small amount and work up gradually to the recommended dosage.

Chamomile
Matricaria recutita

Of the three types of chamomile plant, the most popular and thoroughly studied is German chamomile, used medicinally around the world for thousands of years. Modern herbalists have identified elements in the oil of the chamomile flower that appear to calm the central nervous system, relax the digestive tract and speed healing.

■ TARGET AILMENTS
Take internally for stomach cramps, wind and nervous stomach, indigestion, ulcers, menstrual cramps, insomnia, colic, bladder problems. Use as a gargle for gingivitis and sore throat.
Apply externally for swelling and joint pain, sunburn, cuts and scrapes, teething pain, varicose veins, haemorrhoids.

PREPARATIONS
Over the counter: Available as prepared tea, tincture, essential oil and dried or fresh flowers.
At home:
Tea: Pour 8 fl oz (235 ml) boiling water over 2 tsp chamomile flowers and steep for 10 minutes. Drink this amount three or four times daily.
Fomentation: Apply three or four times daily to sore muscles; sore, swollen joints; varicose veins; and burns and skin wounds.
Herbal bath: Add no more than 2 drops essential oil of chamomile to bathwater.

SIDE EFFECTS
None expected.

SPECIAL INFORMATION
- Allergies to chamomile are rare. However, anyone allergic to other plants in the daisy family should be alert to possible allergic reactions to chamomile.

The 50 Most Effective Herbs

Coltsfoot
Tussilago farfara

Coltsfoot has a long history as a cough suppressant and is still used today for that purpose and as a gentle expectorant. It is banned in Canada, but in the United States the FDA classifies it as an herb with 'undefined safety'. It contains an alkaloid that can seriously damage the liver, and a Japanese study found that the flower buds may be carcinogenic. Many practitioners, however, still routinely use coltsfoot on a short-term basis to treat respiratory ailments.

■ TARGET AILMENTS
Take internally for coughs, asthma and emphysema.
Apply externally for burns, skin ulcers, inflammations and insect bites.

PREPARATIONS
Over the counter: Available in tincture, in capsules and in bulk.
At home:
Tea: Pour 8 fl oz (235 ml) boiling water on to 1 to 3 tsp dried flowers or leaves and steep for 10 minutes. Drink three times a day, as hot as possible.
Compress: Soak a pad in a coltsfoot infusion for several minutes, wring out, then apply to the affected area.
Combinations: For coughs, take it with white horehound and mullein; for bronchitis, with garlic or echinacea.

SIDE EFFECTS
Serious: Fever, nausea, loss of appetite, diarrhoea, jaundice or abdominal pain may result. Stop taking it and call your doctor now.

SPECIAL INFORMATION
WARNING: Use only as prescribed by a practitioner, for short periods of time. Do not give coltsfoot to children under two, pregnant or nursing women, alcoholics or anyone with liver disease.

Dandelion
Taraxacum officinale

Dandelion has a long history of medicinal use. It acts as a natural diuretic while also supplying potassium, a nutrient that is often lost through diuretic use. The plant is rich in vitamins A and C—antioxidants that are believed to help prevent cancer. The young leaves can be eaten fresh or used in herbal preparations.

■ TARGET AILMENTS
Take internally for poor digestion, gallbladder problems, inflammation of the liver. As a supplemental diuretic, dandelion may help relieve symptoms associated with high blood pressure, congestive heart failure, premenstrual syndrome, menstrual pain and joint pain.

PREPARATIONS
Over the counter: Available in tincture, prepared tea, capsule and dried or fresh leaves or roots.
At home:
Tea: Steep 1 tbsp dried or 2 tbsp fresh leaves for each 8 fl oz (235 ml) of boiling water for 10 minutes. Drink up to 32 fl oz (0.9 litre) a day.
Decoction: Simmer 1 tbsp fresh or dried root per 8 fl oz (235 ml) of water for 15 minutes. Drink up to 32 fl oz (0.9 litre) a day.
Nutrition: Add fresh leaves to a salad.

SIDE EFFECTS
Not serious: Allergic dermatitis, stomach upset, diarrhoea, flu-like symptoms, liver pain. Discontinue use and call your doctor.

SPECIAL INFORMATION
❧ Consult a herbalist if you plan to use the herb longer than two or three months, or if you are pregnant, have a heart condition, or suffer from stomach discomfort.
❧ Use low doses for adults over 65 and children between two and 12. Do not give to children under two.

Dong Quai
Angelica sinensis

Also known as Chinese angelica root, dong quai is used by Chinese herbalists as a treatment for several gynaecological complaints. Look for a long, moist, oily plant as the source of the root, which has brown bark and a white cross section. The herb is characterized in traditional Chinese medicine as sweet, acrid, bitter and warm.

■ TARGET AILMENTS
Take internally for menstrual problems; poor blood circulation, pale complexion, possible anaemia; abscesses, sores; lightheadedness, blurred vision, heart palpitations.

PREPARATIONS
This root is available in bulk and in tablet form at health food shops, Asian shops and chemists. You should avoid the herb if it is dry or has a greenish-brown cross-section.

Combinations: Mixed with astragalus, it provides a tonic for treating fatigue. Blend it with white peony root, Chinese foxglove root cooked in wine and cnidium root for menstrual irregularities. Dong quai is also combined with honeysuckle flowers and red peony root to form a preparation that reduces swelling and alleviates pain from abscesses and sores. Consult a Chinese practitioner for further information.

SIDE EFFECTS
None expected if used as directed.

SPECIAL INFORMATION
❧ You should not take dong quai during the early stages of pregnancy.
❧ Check with your Chinese medicine practitioner on the use of this herb if you have diarrhoea or bloating.
❧ Modern acupuncturists sometimes inject the herb into acupuncture points to treat pain, especially that from neuralgia and arthritis.

CONTINUED

The 50 Most Effective Herbs

Echinacea
Echinacea spp.

Echinacea was frequently used by Native Americans of the south-west plains in poultices, mouthwashes, and teas. Now a popular garden perennial, the plant displays purple blossoms and grows as high as 5 ft (1.5 m). Herbalists value the dried root of echinacea for its broad-based action against many types of viral and bacterial illnesses, such as colds, bronchitis, ear infections, influenza and cystitis. Laboratory tests show that echinacea may have antibiotic effects. It seems to bolster the immune system's white blood cells in their battle against foreign microorganisms. It can also be effective as a topical medicine for eczema and other skin problems.

■ TARGET AILMENTS
Take internally for colds, flu, and other respiratory illnesses; glandular fever; ear infections; blood poisoning; bladder infections.
Apply externally for boils, burns, abscesses, wounds, stings, nettle rash, insect bites, eczema, herpes.

PREPARATIONS
Over the counter: Available in tea, capsule, tincture and dried bulk form.
At home:
Tea: Boil 2 tsp dried root in 8 fl oz (235 ml) water and simmer for 15 minutes. Drink three times daily.
Combinations: Use echinacea with yarrow or uva ursi to treat cystitis.

SIDE EFFECTS
None expected.

SPECIAL INFORMATION
⚘ Do not use echinacea continuously for more than a few weeks.
⚘ Do not give to children younger than two; start with minimal doses for older children and older adults.
⚘ Check with your doctor before using if you are pregnant or nursing.

Ephedra
Ephedra sinica

Known in China as ma huang, ephedra has long been used there by healers. Its root and other parts have been used in the West as a decongestant and remedy for asthma, hay fever and colds. Its active ingredients are central nervous system stimulants that open bronchial passages, activating the heart, increasing blood pressure, and speeding up metabolism. For this reason, herbalists warn against excessive use of the herb.

■ TARGET AILMENTS
Take internally for fever, respiratory ailments, hay fever, stomach ache.

PREPARATIONS
Over the counter: Available as fluid extract, tablets, dried bulk herb.
At home:
Chinese: Combine 1 part honey with 4 parts dried herb in a small amount of water. Simmer until water is gone and herbs are slightly brown.
Combinations: For fever and chills, mix with cinnamon twig; for coughing and asthma, with apricot seed; for indigestion, with liquorice.
Western: Boil 1 tsp of the herb with 8 fl oz (235 ml) water for 20 minutes. Drink 16 fl oz (475 ml) a day.

SIDE EFFECTS
Serious: Increased blood pressure or heart rate, heart palpitations. If any of these symptoms develop, discontinue use and consult your doctor immediately.

SPECIAL INFORMATION
WARNING: Because it can cause side effects—and rarely, death—consult a practitioner before taking, especially if you are on any medication. It may not be safe as a weight-loss aid.
WARNING: Do not use if you are pregnant or have heart disease, diabetes, glaucoma or hyperthyroidism.
⚘ Use mild doses for children or seniors. Do not treat children under two.

Eyebright
Euphrasia officinalis

Eyebright is a herb whose name suggests both its action and its appearance. The red spots on its white or purple flowers seem to resemble bloodshot eyes. Moreover, its dried stems, leaves and flowers have long been used as a tonic for irritated or infected eyes. Eyebright can be applied to eyes that are itching, red, and tearing from hay fever, other allergies or colds; it can also alleviate the symptoms of conjunctivitis. Drinking eyebright tea may help to maintain good vision and to diminish nasal congestion and coughs.

■ TARGET AILMENTS
Apply externally for eye irritations from allergies, colds, conjunctivitis.
Take internally for nasal congestion and coughs from colds, sinusitis or allergies.

PREPARATIONS
Over the counter: Available in bulk, capsules and tincture.
At home:
Tea: Pour 8 fl oz (235 ml) boiling water on to 2 tsp dried herb and steep for 10 minutes; drink 3 times daily.
Compress: Boil 1 to 2 tbsp dried eyebright in 16 fl oz (475 ml) water for 10 minutes. After this has cooled, strain it, dip a sterile cloth in it and wring it out, then put it on your eyes for 15 minutes a few times a day.
Combinations to be taken orally: For congestion, combine it with goldenrod, elder flowers or goldenseal. For hay fever, mix it with ephedra. Consult a herbalist for dosages.

SIDE EFFECTS
Not serious: Eyebright may cause a skin rash or nausea. If this occurs, lessen your dose or stop taking completely.

SPECIAL INFORMATION
⚘ Consult a practitioner before using eyebright to treat children.

The 50 Most Effective Herbs

Feverfew

Tanacetum parthenium
(or *Chrysanthemum parthenium*)

Feverfew is a perennial with small-blossoms that resemble daisies. In the late 1970s British researchers found feverfew leaves helpful in treating migraine headaches where other treatments had failed. They believe this relief is due to the chemical parthenolide, which blocks the release of inflammatory substances from the blood. The researchers consider these inflammatory elements to be key components in the onset of a migraine.

■ TARGET AILMENTS
Take internally for migraines.

PREPARATIONS
Over the counter: Available in dry bulk, pills, capsules and tinctures.
At home: Chew two fresh or frozen leaves a day for migraines. If you find the leaves too bitter, substitute capsules or pills containing 85 mg of the leaf material, but fresh leaves are best for immediate results.

Tea: Steep 2 tsp dried herb in 8 fl oz (235 ml) boiling water for 5–10 minutes; drink 16–24 fl oz (475–700 ml) per day.

SIDE EFFECTS
Serious: Chewing fresh or dried feverfew may cause internal mouth sores or abdominal pain. If these symptoms develop, discontinue use and notify your doctor.

SPECIAL INFORMATION
- Do not take if you are pregnant.
- Feverfew may interfere with the blood's clotting ability; talk to your doctor before using if you have a clotting disorder or take anticoagulant medicine.
- You may need to take feverfew daily for two to three months before it has any effect.

Garlic

Allium sativum

The garlic bulb has long been recognized as a medicinal remedy in Chinese and Western cultures. Garlic's active ingredient is allicin, which is also responsible for the herb's pungent smell. In China this herb is prescribed for colds and coughs and for intestinal and digestive disorders. Chinese herbalists believe garlic can be used externally as an antibiotic and anti-fungal treatment for skin infections. Western herbalists prescribe it for many of the same ailments as their Chinese counterparts. It is also used to reduce cholesterol and to lower blood pressure.

■ TARGET AILMENTS
Take internally for colds, coughs, flu, high cholesterol, high blood pressure, atherosclerosis, digestive disorders, bladder infection, liver and gallbladder problems.
Apply externally for athlete's foot, ringworm, minor skin infections.

PREPARATIONS
Over the counter: Garlic is available as cloves and in tablet form.
At home:
Tincture: Combine 8 fl oz (235 ml) crushed cloves with 64 fl oz (1.9 litres) brandy. Shake daily for two weeks. Take up to 3 tbsp a day.

SIDE EFFECTS
Not serious: Allergic rash from touching or eating the herb.

SPECIAL INFORMATION
- Consult your practitioner before using garlic if you are pregnant.
- Garlic has a blood clot-preventing agent. If you have a blood-clotting disorder, consult a herbalist or a doctor
- Garlic is thought to function as an adjunct treatment for cardiovascular disease. Consult your doctor before using it in this capacity.

Ginger

Zingiber officinale

Ginger not only is a valued culinary seasoning but also is considered a remedy for a range of ailments. Both Chinese and Western herbalists believe it relieves motion sickness and dizziness and improves digestion. Ginger is also said to alleviate menstrual cramps. Its active constituents, gingerols, soothe the abdomen and relieve excess wind In China, ginger, called gan-jian, is applied to first- and second-degree burns.

■ TARGET AILMENTS
Chinese: vomiting, abdominal pain, menstrual irregularity (take internally); minor burns (apply externally).
Western: motion sickness, digestive disorders, menstrual cramps, colds, flu, arthritis, high cholesterol, high blood pressure (take internally).

PREPARATIONS
Over the counter: Available as fresh or dried root, liquid extract, tablets, capsules, prepared tea.
At home:
Chinese: Wrap fresh roots in five or six layers of rice paper. Bury under warm coals until the paper is blackened. Discard paper before use.
Rub: Treat minor burns by rubbing fresh ginger juice on the wound.
Combinations: For vomiting, mix with pinellia root; when there is also severe abdominal pain, combine with liquorice or galanga. A preparation of ginger and chamomile is used to treat menstrual irregularity.
Western: Boil 1 oz (30 g) dried root in 8 fl oz (235 ml) water for 15 to 20 minutes for tea.

SIDE EFFECTS
Not serious: Heartburn.

SPECIAL INFORMATION
- Ginger may help prevent heart disease and strokes.
- If you are pregnant, consult your doctor before using.

CONTINUED

The 50 Most Effective Herbs

Ginkgo
Ginkgo biloba

Chinese herbalists have used the fan-shaped leaves of the ginkgo tree for thousands of years to treat asthma, chilblains and swelling. Western herbalists value it for its action against vascular diseases. It dilates blood vessels and thereby improves blood flow, especially to areas such as the lower legs and feet, as well as to the brain. Herbalists believe ginkgo can keep blood clots from forming and bronchial tubes from constricting during an asthma attack. It may also help reduce damage from macular degeneration.

■ **TARGET AILMENTS**
Take internally for vertigo; tinnitus; phlebitis; leg ulcers; cerebral atherosclerosis; diabetic vascular disease; Raynaud's syndrome; headache; depression; lack of concentration or mental and emotional fatigue in the elderly; asthma; clotting disorders, including stroke and heart attack.

PREPARATIONS
Leaves are available in dry bulk, capsules or tincture. You can find ginkgo biloba extract (GBE) in health food shops. Most herbalists recommend using only over-the-counter ginkgo products.

SIDE EFFECTS
Not serious: Irritability, restlessness, diarrhoea, nausea; check with your doctor to see if you should lower your dose or stop taking it completely.

SPECIAL INFORMATION
WARNING: Some people cannot tolerate ginkgo even in small doses.
🍃 Do not use if you have a bleeding disorder such as haemophilia or are pregnant or nursing.
🍃 Do not give ginkgo to children without a doctor's supervision.
🍃 Consult a doctor before using it in medicinal amounts.

Ginseng, American
Panax quinquefolius

Native Americans believed American ginseng could alleviate painful childbirths and restore energy in the elderly. American ginseng is identified by a single stalk crowned by delicate chartreuse blooms and crimson berries; its leaflets have saw-like teeth. The active ingredients of American ginseng are panaxosides, which are thought to calm the stomach and the brain and act as a mild stimulant to vital organs. American ginseng is milder than Asian ginseng and is often prescribed for people who consider Asian ginseng too potent. Both American and Asian ginseng are frequently used to treat the elderly.

■ **TARGET AILMENTS**
Take internally for depression, fatigue, stress, colds, influenza, respiratory problems, inflammation, a damaged immune system.

PREPARATIONS
Over the counter: Ginseng is available as fresh or dried root, root powder, capsules, tablets, prepared tea, freeze-dried root, cured sweets.
At home:
Decoction: Boil 1 oz (30 g) fresh root with 8 fl oz (235 ml) water for 15 to 20 minutes. Drink up to 16 fl oz (475 ml) a day.

SIDE EFFECTS
Not serious: Headache, insomnia, anxiety, breast soreness, skin rash.
Serious: You may experience asthma attacks, increased blood pressure, heart palpitations, or post-menopausal uterine bleeding. Discontinue use of ginseng and consult your doctor.

Ginseng, Asian
Panax ginseng

Growing in the mountains of north-east China, Asian ginseng is the most potent and expensive form of ginseng. With its yellow-green flowers and red berries, it looks like American ginseng, but the stalk is longer. Its active constituents are ginsenosides, substances that strengthen the immune system and increase the body's ability to deal with fatigue and stress. Herbalists prescribe Asian ginseng root for fever, colds, coughs and menstrual irregularities.

■ **TARGET AILMENTS**
Take internally for depression, fatigue, stress, colds, flu, respiratory problems, inflammation, a damaged immune system.

PREPARATIONS
Over the counter: Ginseng is available as fresh or dried root, root powder, capsules, tablets, prepared tea, freeze-dried root, cured sweets.
At home:
Decoction: Boil 1 oz (30 g) fresh root with 8 fl oz (235 ml) water for 15 to 20 minutes. Drink up to 16 fl oz (475 ml) a day.

SIDE EFFECTS
Not serious: Headache, insomnia, anxiety, breast soreness or skin rash.
Serious: Asthma attacks, increased blood pressure, heart palpitations or post-menopausal uterine bleeding. Stop using ginseng and consult your doctor.

SPECIAL INFORMATION
🍃 Use only under the direction of a herbalist or doctor if you are pregnant or have insomnia, hay fever, fibrocystic breasts, asthma, emphysema, high blood pressure, blood-clotting or heart disorders or diabetes.

The 50 Most Effective Herbs

Goldenseal
Hydrastis canadensis

Herbalists use the dried and powdered rhizomes and roots of the perennial goldenseal to treat several respiratory and skin infections. The herb acts as a stimulant and seems to affect the body's mucous membranes by drying up secretions, reducing inflammation and fighting infection. Goldenseal also aids digestion and may control postpartum bleeding.

■ **TARGET AILMENTS**

Take internally for stomach problems; sore throat; infected gums, ears and sinuses; postpartum bleeding.

Apply externally for eczema, ringworm, contact dermatitis, athlete's foot, impetigo.

PREPARATIONS

Over the counter: Dry root is available in bulk, capsules and tincture.

At home:

Tea: Pour 8 fl oz (235 ml) boiling water on to 2 tsp goldenseal; steep for 10–15 minutes. Drink 3 times daily.

Combinations: Use with meadowsweet and chamomile for stomach problems. For a skin wash, mix with distilled witch hazel; for ear infections, make drops using goldenseal and mullein. See your herbalist for exact instructions.

SIDE EFFECTS

Not serious: In high doses, it can irritate the skin, mouth, and throat and cause nausea and diarrhoea. If any of these develop, stop taking it.

SPECIAL INFORMATION

❧ Do not take if you are pregnant.

❧ Do not use goldenseal without consulting a doctor if you have had heart disease, diabetes, glaucoma, a stroke or high blood pressure.

❧ Do not give goldenseal to children under two; for older children and older adults, start with small doses.

Gotu Kola
Centella asiatica

The gotu kola plant grows in marshy areas in many parts of the world. Its fan-shaped leaves contain the soothing agent known as asiaticoside. As a result they have been used to treat burns, skin grafts and episiotomies. Gotu kola may also help heal outbreaks of psoriasis and may help decrease oedema and promote blood circulation in the legs. It may therefore be useful in treating phlebitis.

■ **TARGET AILMENTS**

Take internally for poor circulation in the legs, oedema.

Apply externally for burns, cuts, and other skin injuries; psoriasis. (Use a compress.)

PREPARATIONS

Over the counter: Available in dry bulk, capsules and tincture.

At home:

Tea: Use 1 to 2 tsp dried gotu kola per 8 fl oz (235 ml) of boiling water; drink twice daily to improve circulation.

Compress: Soak a pad in a tea or in a tincture to help treat wounds or psoriasis. Start with a weak solution and increase the concentration of gotu kola if necessary.

SIDE EFFECTS

Not serious: Gotu kola may cause a skin rash or headaches; in either case, lower your dosage or stop taking it.

SPECIAL INFORMATION

❧ Do not use gotu kola if you are pregnant or nursing, or using tranquillizers or sedatives, since gotu kola may have a narcotic effect.

❧ Do not give gotu kola to children under two. For older children and older adults, start with low-strength doses and increase if necessary.

Hawthorn
Crataegus laevigata (or C. oxyacantha)

Herbalists use the flowers, fruit and leaves of the hawthorn, a European shrub with thorny branches. They prescribe the herb as a mild heart tonic. It is thought to dilate the blood vessels, thereby facilitating the flow of blood in the arteries and lowering blood pressure. Hawthorn is also believed to increase the pumping force of the heart muscle and to eliminate arrhythmias. It may have a calming effect on the nervous system and is sometimes recommended as a remedy for insomnia.

■ **TARGET AILMENTS**

Take internally in conjunction with conventional medical treatment for high blood pressure, clogged arteries, heart palpitations, angina, inflammation of the heart muscle.

Take internally for insomnia and nervous conditions. Use as a gargle for sore throat.

PREPARATIONS

Hawthorn is available as fluid extract, dried berries and leaves, capsules.

SIDE EFFECTS

Serious: Taking large amounts of hawthorn may result in a dramatic drop in blood pressure, which in turn may cause you to feel faint.

SPECIAL INFORMATION

WARNING: Use hawthorn as a heart tonic only if you have been diagnosed with angina, cardiac arrhythmias or congestive heart failure, and only in consultation with a doctor. Do not practice self-diagnosis.

❧ Children and pregnant or nursing women should use hawthorn only under the direction of a medical herbalist or doctor.

CONTINUED

The 50 Most Effective Herbs

Horsetail
Equisetum arvense

Horsetail has been valued since ancient times for its ability to stem the flow of blood, bind tissues and increase urine production. It is rich in silica, which helps mend broken bones and form collagen. Herbalists today prescribe horsetail for wounds, urinary problems, benign prostate disorders and the pain of rheumatism or arthritis.

■ **TARGET AILMENTS**
Take internally for bladder and kidney problems, prostatitis, ulcers; broken bones or sprains; strengthening bones and nails; joint pain.
Apply externally for sores and inflammation.

PREPARATIONS
Over the counter: Available dried or fresh, in capsules and in tincture.
At home:
Tea: Steep 2 tsp dried or 1 tbsp fresh herb per 8 fl oz (235 ml) boiling water for 15 minutes. Drink cold, up to 32 fl oz (0.9 litre) a day, 2 tbsp at a time. Apply to cuts.
Combinations: Use with hydrangea for prostate problems.

SIDE EFFECTS
Not serious: Upset stomach, diarrhoea, increased urination. Discontinue and call your doctor.
Serious: Kidney or lower back pain, or pain on urination; cardiac problems. Call your doctor now.

SPECIAL INFORMATION
WARNING: Do not take for more than three days in a row, and follow the given dosage; extended use may cause kidney or cardiac damage.
⮞ Use only under a doctor's care. Heart disease or high blood pressure patients should use with caution.
⮞ Use mild doses for adults over 65 and children aged 2–12. Children under 2 and pregnant women should not use horsetail.

Hyssop
Hyssopus officinalis

Hyssop, a member of the mint family, is used as an expectorant, digestive aid, sedative and muscle relaxant. It is also used as an antiseptic; its oils may heal wounds and herpes simplex sores.

■ **TARGET AILMENTS**
Take internally for coughs, colds, bronchitis; indigestion, wind; anxiety, hysteria; petit mal seizures.
Apply externally for cold sores, genital herpes sores, burns, wounds, skin irritations.

PREPARATIONS
Over the counter: Available dried or fresh and as tincture.
At home:
Tea: Steep 2 tsp dried herb per cup of boiling water for 10 to 15 minutes. Drink three times a day for cough; gargle three times a day for sore throat. Apply to burns and wounds.
Compress: Steep 1 oz dried herb in 16 fl oz (475 ml) boiling water for 15 minutes; soak clean cloth in solution and apply warm to cold sores or genital herpes sores; place on the chest to relieve congestion.
Combinations: Used with white horehound and coltsfoot for coughs and bronchitis; with boneset, elder flower and peppermint for cold symptoms; and with sage as a gargle for sore throats.

SIDE EFFECTS
Not serious: Upset stomach. Discontinue and call a doctor.

SPECIAL INFORMATION
⮞ Use hyssop only under medical supervision if you use it for more than three consecutive days.
⮞ Do not use hyssop if pregnant; it was once used to induce abortion.
⮞ Use low-strength preparations for adults over 65 or children between two and 12 years of age. Do not give to children under two years old.

Juniper
Juniperus communis

Juniper acts as a diuretic and thus is used to treat high blood pressure and PMS. Juniper oil is thought to have anti-inflammatory effects useful for treating arthritis and gout. Juniper teas can be taken for digestive problems.

■ **TARGET AILMENTS**
Take internally for bladder infections, cystitis, oedema; digestive problems; menstrual irregularities and PMS; high blood pressure.
Apply externally for arthritis, gout.

PREPARATIONS
Over the counter: Available in whole berries, bulk, and capsules, and as tincture.
At home:
Tea: Steep 1 tsp ground juniper berries in 8 fl oz (235 ml) boiling water for 10 to 20 minutes. Drink at least two times daily. Do not use for more than six weeks at a time.

SIDE EFFECTS
Not serious: Individuals with hay fever may develop allergy symptoms such as nasal congestion when taking juniper. If this happens, stop taking the herb and call your doctor.
Serious: Juniper in high doses can irritate and damage the kidneys and urinary tract. If you develop diarrhoea, intestinal pain, kidney pain, blood in the urine, purplish urine or a faster heartbeat, stop taking juniper immediately and see your doctor as soon as possible.

SPECIAL INFORMATION
WARNING: Because it can irritate the kidneys and urinary tract, juniper is suitable for short-term use only.
WARNING: Do not use juniper if you have or have had kidney problems.
⮞ Pregnant women should not use juniper, because it may stimulate contraction of the uterus.

The 50 Most Effective Herbs

Kelp
Fucus spp.

Extracts of iodine-rich kelp, one of the many forms of seaweed, provided an effective goitre remedy for many years. Today some herbalists rely on another component of kelp's stem-like and leaf-like parts, an agent known as sodium alginate. Because of its action, kelp is prescribed to aid in the treatment of heavy-metal environmental pollutants, including barium and cadmium, and to prevent the body from absorbing strontium 90, a radioactive substance created in nuclear power plants.

Some practitioners of alternative medicine also recommend taking kelp supplements for thyroid disorders such as mild hypothyroidism (underactive thyroid).

■ TARGET AILMENTS
Take internally for goitre, hypothyroidism, radiation exposure, heavy-metal environmental pollutants.

PREPARATIONS
Over the counter: Available in dry bulk, capsules and tincture.
At home:
Infusion: Steep 2 to 3 tsp dried or powdered kelp in 8 fl oz (235 ml) boiling water for 10 minutes; drink three times daily.

SIDE EFFECTS
None expected.

SPECIAL INFORMATION
WARNING: If you are already taking medication for hyperthyroidism (overactive thyroid), kelp supplements could worsen the condition.
WARNING: Do not gather your own wild kelp for use; coastal colonies may be contaminated by offshore pollutants.
WARNING: Check with your practitioner before using kelp if you have a history of thyroid problems or high blood pressure.

Lavender
Lavandula officinalis

A fragrant herb that scents clothes and helps repel moths, lavender also has medicinal properties. Herbalists prescribe lavender tea and the essential oil of lavender, both made from the plant's flowers, to treat common minor ailments such as insomnia, headache, and nausea. Anecdotal evidence suggests that lavender has a calming effect that relieves anxiety and promotes gastrointestinal relaxation. Its aroma (particularly that of L. angustifolia) is thought to stimulate mental processes and help alleviate depression, especially when it is used with other herbs. Like many aromatic essential oils, lavender oil has antiseptic qualities that may kill several types of disease-causing bacteria, and herbalists use it to treat skin ailments such as fungus, burns, wounds and eczema.

■ TARGET AILMENTS
Take internally for insomnia, depression, or headache, especially when caused by stress; poor digestion, nausea, flatulence, colic.
Apply externally for burns, wounds, eczema, acne, candidiasis, ringworm, rheumatism.

PREPARATIONS
Over the counter: Available in dried bulk, capsules, oil and tincture.
At home:
Tea: Steep 1 tsp dried flowers in 8 fl oz (235 ml) boiling water for 10 minutes; drink three times daily.
Oil: To relax, use a few drops of the essential oil in a bath; rub it on your skin to ease rheumatic pains; or use a few drops in a steam inhalation for coughs, colds, and flu.
Combinations: For depression, lavender can be used with rosemary, skullcap or kola.

SPECIAL INFORMATION
WARNING: Do not use oil of lavender internally.

Liquorice
Glycyrrhiza glabra

Liquorice is one of the most common medicinal herbs. Its intense sweetness masks the bitterness of herbal mixtures. Chinese and Western herbalists use liquorice root as a cough suppressant and for digestive disorders, believing that it acts as a mild laxative and prevents stomach ulcers by forming a protective coating on the stomach wall. Practitioners think that liquorice, as an external antibiotic, relieves skin irritations such as eczema and herpes sores.

■ TARGET AILMENTS
Take internally for cough, sore throat, colic, constipation, heartburn, stomach ulcers, arthritis, hepatitis, cirrhosis.
Apply externally for skin infections, eczema, herpes sores.

PREPARATIONS
Over the counter: Available as dried root, liquid extract and capsules.
At home:
Tea: Prepare by boiling 1 oz (30 g) liquorice root in 8 fl oz (235 ml) water for 15 to 20 minutes. Drink up to twice this amount daily.
Antibiotic: Sprinkle liquorice powder directly on the infection or sore.

SIDE EFFECTS
Not serious: Upset stomach, diarrhoea, headache, oedema (fluid retention), grogginess, weakness.

SPECIAL INFORMATION
WARNING: Large amounts taken over a long period can lead to high blood pressure and oedema. Consult your practitioner for advice.
≉ Do not use liquorice root if you have oedema, high blood pressure, kidney disease or glaucoma.
≉ Avoid the herb if you are pregnant. It increases production of aldosterone, a hormone that regulates the salt and water balance in the body, resulting in a rise in blood pressure.

CONTINUED

The 50 Most Effective Herbs

Lobelia
Lobelia inflata

Lobelia, sometimes called Indian tobacco, is prescribed for both respiratory ailments and external conditions, but it can be extremely toxic. Because it is thought to relax overworked bronchial muscles and promote coughing, lobelia is most widely used to treat respiratory illnesses. Lobelia compresses have been used to treat skin injuries, fungus infections and muscle strains.

■ TARGET AILMENTS
Take internally for pneumonia, asthma, bronchitis.
Apply externally for bruises, insect bites, fungus infections including ringworm, muscle strains.

PREPARATIONS
Over the counter: Available in dried bulk, capsules and tincture.
At home:
Tea: Steep ¼–½ tsp dried leaves in 8 fl oz (235 ml) boiling water for 10–15 minutes; drink three times daily.
Compress: Soak a piece of cloth in an infusion for several minutes; wring out and apply to affected area.
Combinations: For asthma, use with cayenne, skunk cabbage and ginger.

SIDE EFFECTS
Serious:
WARNING: Lobelia poisoning can cause nausea, excessive salivation, diarrhoea, impaired hearing and vision, weakness, and mental confusion, and if not treated promptly can bring on respiratory failure and even death. If you develop any side effects, call your doctor at once.

SPECIAL INFORMATION
WARNING: Use lobelia only in doses prescribed by your practitioner.
❧ If your practitioner prescribes lobelia for your child, monitor the child frequently for the development of any side effects.

Marsh Mallow
Althaea officinalis

For centuries people in Europe and the Middle East have eaten wild-growing marsh mallow when their crops failed. Today it is still recognized as a wilderness forage food. Herbalists use the roots, and sometimes the leaves, to treat cuts and wounds, mouth sores, stomach distress and other ailments. And teething, irritable babies and toddlers have traditionally found comfort in sucking on a root of marsh mallow.

The healing substance in marsh mallow is mucilage, a spongy root material that forms a gel when mixed with water and is especially soothing to inflamed mucous membranes. One study suggests that mucilage supports the immune system's white blood cells in their fight against invading microbes. Another trial indicates that marsh mallow may help to lower blood sugar.

■ TARGET AILMENTS
Take internally for sore throat, coughs, colds, flu, bronchitis, sinusitis; upset stomach, peptic ulcers, gastritis, colitis; cystitis, bladder infections, urethritis, kidney stones.
Apply externally for abscesses, boils, skin ulcers, scrapes, cuts, burns, other wounds; varicose veins; dental abscesses, gingivitis.

PREPARATIONS
Over the counter: Available in dried bulk, capsules, tincture.
At home:
Decoction: Simmer 1–2 tsp finely chopped or crushed root in 8 fl oz (235 ml) water for 10–15 minutes; drink 3 times daily. Use this as a gargle for mouth problems.
Gel: Add just enough water to the finely chopped root to give it a gel-like consistency and use for skin problems.

SPECIAL INFORMATION
❧ Marsh mallow can be given in low doses to infants and children.

Milk Thistle
Silybum marianum

Milk thistle is used by herbalists to treat such liver disorders as cirrhosis and hepatitis. The active ingredient, silymarin, found in the seeds, is believed to prompt the growth of new, healthy liver cells without encouraging any malignancy that may be present. It is also thought that silymarin acts as an antioxidant, protecting the liver from damage by free radicals, harmful by-products of many bodily processes. The use of silymarin by healthy people can greatly increase the liver's content of glutathione, a key agent in detoxifying many potentially harmful substances.

Milk thistle also is believed to ease outbreaks of psoriasis, since these may worsen when the liver fails to neutralize certain toxins.

■ TARGET AILMENTS
Take internally for liver problems; inflammation of the gallbladder duct; psoriasis.

PREPARATIONS
Over the counter: Available in dried bulk, capsules, extract.
At home:
Tea: Steep 1 tsp freshly ground seeds in 8 fl oz (235 ml) boiling water for 10 to 15 minutes; drink three times daily. Or eat 1 tsp of freshly ground seeds. Milk thistle extract may be more effective than teas, since silymarin is only slightly water soluble. See a herbalist for more information.

SIDE EFFECTS
Not serious: Because taking milk thistle increases bile secretion, you may develop loose stools.

SPECIAL INFORMATION
WARNING: If you think you have a liver disorder, seek medical advice.

Mugwort Leaf
Artemisia argyi (or A. vulgaris)

Mugwort leaf is prescribed in Chinese medicine for a range of gynaecological problems. In China mugwort is harvested at the end of spring or in early summer, when the leaves are growing vigorously but the flowers have not yet bloomed. The best leaves are greyish white with a thick, hairy texture. In Western tradition it is used to aid digestion and combat depression.

■ **TARGET AILMENTS**
Take internally for excessive menstrual bleeding and cramps, uterine bleeding, vaginal pain and bleeding during pregnancy, threatened miscarriage; a digestive aid; depression.

PREPARATIONS
Leaves are available in bulk at some health food and Asian shops and chemists. The herb is also sold in pills. The dried, aged, powdered herb can be rolled in tissue paper into a cigar-like cylinder; one end is burned near the site of an injury to increase blood circulation and relieve pain. Acupuncturists sometimes use this technique instead of inserting needles.

Combinations: A mixture with gelatin is prescribed for vaginal bleeding and pain during pregnancy or for spotting between periods. Combining mugwort with dried ginger targets menstrual pain. And a preparation of mugwort leaves and kochia fruit is applied to itching lesions on the skin. For information on dosages and other preparations, check with a herbal practitioner.

SIDE EFFECTS
None expected.

SPECIAL INFORMATION
❧ A clinical trial suggests that crushed fresh leaves may eradicate warts.
❧ The herb seems to indicate an antibiotic effect in test-tube studies.

Mullein
Verbascum thapsus

Mullein is useful in treating diarrhoea and haemorrhoids and, as an expectorant, bronchitis and coughs.

■ **TARGET AILMENTS**
Take internally for respiratory ailments; gastrointestinal problems (stomach cramps, diarrhoea.).
Apply externally for external ulcers, tumours, haemorrhoids.

PREPARATIONS
Over the counter: Mullein is available as tincture and as dried leaves, flowers, or roots.
At home:
Tea: Steep 1 to 2 tsp dried leaves, flowers, or roots per 8 fl oz (235 ml) of boiling water for 10 or 15 minutes. Drink as much as 3 times this amount a day.
Compress: Soak bandages in a cooled tea made with vinegar; apply to ulcers, tumours or haemorrhoids.
Inhalant: Boil fresh leaves in water and inhale the steam to relieve coughs and congestion.
Combinations: With elder and red clover for painful coughing; with gumweed for asthma; as an extract in olive oil for external ulcers, haemorrhoids, tumours; with white horehound, coltsfoot and lobelia for bronchitis.

SIDE EFFECTS
Not serious: Mild stomach upset or diarrhoea. Reduce dosage or discontinue; consult your doctor when convenient.

SPECIAL INFORMATION
WARNING: If you have a history of cancer, consult your doctor before ingesting this herb; the tannin in mullein may be carcinogenic.
WARNING: Do not ingest the seeds; they are toxic.
WARNING: Do not take mullein if you are pregnant or nursing a baby.

Nettle
Urtica dioica

Notorious for its stinging needles, nettle can be safely ingested when boiled or dried. Herbalists consider nettle a diuretic capable of removing toxins. Nettle has an erect stem and serrated, heart-shaped, dark green leaves.

■ **TARGET AILMENTS**
Take internally for arthritis, gout, hay fever, premenstrual syndrome, vaginal yeast infections, excessive menstrual flow, haemorrhoids, eczema, diarrhoea, chronic cystitis.
Take internally only under a doctor's supervision for high blood pressure, congestive heart failure.

PREPARATIONS
Over the counter: Nettle is available as tincture, capsules, and dried leaves and stems.
At home:
Tea: Steep 1–2 tsp dried herb in 8 fl oz (235 ml) boiling water for 10 mins. Drink up to twice this a day.
Juice: Add 2 tsp juice squeezed from nettle to a vegetable or fruit drink.
Combinations: Nettle combines well with figwort and burdock to treat eczema; take orally as juice or tea.

SIDE EFFECTS
Not serious: Large doses of nettle tea may cause stomach irritation, constipation, burning skin or urinary suppression. Stop taking the herb and call your doctor.

SPECIAL INFORMATION
WARNING: Do not use uncooked nettle; it may cause kidney damage and other symptoms of poisoning.
WARNING: Nettle is a diuretic, and it may therefore remove potassium from the body. If you use it frequently, eat foods high in potassium.
❧ Do not give nettle to children younger than two years old.
❧ To harvest, wear gloves and long sleeves to avoid the sting.

CONTINUED

Parsley

Petroselinum crispum

Added to foods or used as a garnish, parsley leaves are a source of vitamins C and A, as well as a versatile herbal remedy. Because it eases muscle spasms and cramps, parsley is used as a digestive aid, and it is prescribed as a diuretic and mild laxative. Parsley is also considered to be an expectorant.

■ TARGET AILMENTS

Take internally for indigestion, congestion from coughs and colds, asthma, irregular menstruation, premenstrual syndrome, fever.

Take internally under a doctor's supervision for high blood pressure, congestive heart failure.

PREPARATIONS

Over the counter: Available as tincture and as fresh or dried leaves, seeds, stems and roots.

At home:
Tea: Steep 1 to 2 tsp dried leaves or roots per 8 fl oz (235 ml) of boiling water for 5 to 10 minutes in a closed container. Drink up to 3 times this a day.
Nutrition and diet: Eat raw green leaves as a breath freshener.

SIDE EFFECTS
None expected.

SPECIAL INFORMATION
WARNING: Pregnant and nursing women should not take parsley juice or oil in medicinal doses. Eating a few sprigs served as garnish will probably not cause any harm.
WARNING: If you use this herb frequently as a medicine, you should also eat foods high in potassium, such as bananas, because diuretics deplete the body of potassium.
☙ Do not give medicinal doses to children younger than two years old.
☙ Only experienced field botanists should pick wild parsley, because of its resemblance to toxic plants.

Passionflower

Passiflora incarnata

Because of its purported calming effect on the central nervous system, herbalists use passionflower as a sedative, a digestive aid and a pain reliever.

■ TARGET AILMENTS
Take internally for insomnia, anxiety, neuralgia, shingles, persistent hiccups, asthma, and to aid withdrawal from addictive disorders.

PREPARATIONS
Over the counter: Available in commercial homoeopathic or herbal remedies and as dried or fresh leaves, capsules, and tincture.
At home:
Tea: Steep 2 tsp dried herb per 8 fl oz (235 ml) of boiling water for 15 minutes. For insomnia, drink this amount in the evening.
Tincture: 1 dropperful in warm water, up to 4 times a day, for anxiety in adults and in children over 100 lb (45 kg). Give to smaller children only under medical supervision.

SIDE EFFECTS
Not serious: Gastric upset, diarrhoea. Discontinue and call your doctor.
Serious: May cause sleepiness; do not take during the day if you operate heavy machinery or drive.

SPECIAL INFORMATION
☙ Always use passionflower under medical supervision.
☙ Use only professionally prepared remedies; another species, *Passiflora caerulea*, contains cyanide.
☙ Do not take if you are pregnant.
☙ Use low-strength preparations for adults over 65 or children between two and 12 years old. Do not give to children under two years of age.

POSSIBLE INTERACTIONS
Use caution when combining with prescription sedatives.

Pau d'Arco

Tabebuia impetiginosa

Pau d'arco is the name of both a tree and a medicinal extract from the tree's bark or heartwood. The extract is believed to be effective against bacterial, fungal, viral and parasitic infections, and is also considered to be an anti-inflammatory agent. It is thought to destroy microorganisms by increasing the supply of oxygen to cells. For centuries before modern science isolated some 20 of its chemical ingredients, pau d'arco was used as a folk remedy. The pau d'arco tree, also called the trumpet tree, is native to Central and South America and the West Indies. It can reach a height of 125 ft (38 m).

■ TARGET AILMENTS
Take internally for bacterial, fungal, viral and parasitic infections; indigestion.

PREPARATIONS
Over the counter: Pau d'arco is available as capsules, tincture and dried bark.
At home:
Decoction: Boil 1 tbsp bark in 16–24 fl oz (475–700 ml) water for 10 to 15 minutes. Drink 16–64 fl oz (475 ml–1.9 litre) a day.

SIDE EFFECTS
None expected.

The 50 Most Effective Herbs

Peppermint
Mentha piperita

Peppermint plants have stems with a purplish cast; long, serrated leaves; and a familiar minty aroma. This common, pleasant-tasting herb has been used as a remedy for indigestion since the time of the pharaohs of ancient Egypt. Menthol, the principal active ingredient, stimulates the stomach lining, thereby reducing the amount of time food spends in the stomach. It also relaxes the muscles of the digestive system.

■ **TARGET AILMENTS**
Take internally for cramps, stomach pain, wind, nausea associated with migraine headaches, morning sickness, travel sickness, insomnia, anxiety, fever, colds, flu.
Apply externally for itching and inflammation.

PREPARATIONS
Over the counter: Available as commercial tea, tincture and fresh or dried leaves and flowers.
At home:
Tea: Drink commercial brands or steep 1 to 2 heaping tsp dried herb per 8 fl oz (235 ml) of boiling water for 10 minutes. Drink up to 24 fl oz (0.7 litre) a day.
Bath: Fill a cloth bag with several handfuls of dried or fresh herb and let hot water run over it.

SIDE EFFECTS
None expected.

SPECIAL INFORMATION
WARNING: Do not ingest pure menthol or pure peppermint; these substances are extremely toxic.
⚬ Give only very dilute preparations to children younger than two and only under a doctor's supervision.
⚬ Pregnant women with morning sickness should use a dilute tea rather than a more potent infusion. Peppermint should not be used by women who have a history of miscarriage.

Psyllium
Plantago psyllium

Psyllium, whose fibre-rich seeds make a safe, bulk-forming laxative, has long been used to treat constipation, diarrhoea, haemorrhoids and urinary problems. Because the herb absorbs excess fluid in the intestinal tract and increases stool volume, both diarrhoea and constipation can be treated.

■ **TARGET AILMENTS**
Take internally for constipation, haemorrhoidal irritation, diarrhoea.

PREPARATIONS
Over the counter: Available as whole seeds, ground or powdered seeds, and in various commercial bulk-forming laxative preparations.
At home:
Drink: Mix 1 tsp ground seeds or powder in 8 fl oz (235 ml) cool liquid. Drink 16–24 fl oz (475–700 ml) a day.
Seeds: Take 1 tsp seeds with water at mealtimes.

SIDE EFFECTS
Not serious: Psyllium can cause allergic reactions in people who have allergies to dust or grasses. Call your doctor if bothersome.
Serious: Severe allergic reactions are rare; if you have difficulty breathing, seek emergency help.

SPECIAL INFORMATION
WARNING: To prevent intestinal blockage when taking psyllium as a laxative, you must drink 8 to 10 glasses of water throughout the day.
⚬ Start using this herb gradually to allow your body to adjust to the increase in fibre.
⚬ Do not give this herb to children younger than two years of age. Consult your doctor if your infant or child is constipated.
⚬ If you are pregnant, avoid psyllium and all laxatives because they stimulate the lower pelvis.

Red Clover
Trifolium pratense

The medicinal parts of this perennial are the red or purple ball-shaped flowers. Herbalists prescribe red clover for skin ailments, indigestion and coughs. It is an anti-inflammatory agent and, as an expectorant, helps remove excess mucus from the lungs. In addition, the herb appears to act like the female hormone oestrogen; it is believed to help women with menopausal symptoms.

■ **TARGET AILMENTS**
Take internally for coughs, bronchitis, whooping cough, indigestion, menopausal symptoms.
Use internally and externally for skin problems such as eczema and psoriasis.

PREPARATIONS
Over the counter: Red clover is available in dried bulk and tincture.
At home:
Tea: Steep 1 to 3 tsp dried flower tops in 8 fl oz (235 ml) boiling water for 15 minutes. Drink up to 3 times this amount daily.
Compress: Soak a clean cloth in the infusion and apply to the skin.

SIDE EFFECTS
Serious: Discontinue use if you experience stomach aches or diarrhoea.

SPECIAL INFORMATION
WARNING: Do not use red clover if you are pregnant, because of its oestrogen-like behaviour.
WARNING: Avoid the herb if you have oestrogen-dependent cancer or a history of heart disease, stroke or thrombophlebitis.
⚬ If you are taking birth control pills, consult your doctor before using red clover.
⚬ Do not give the herb to children under two. Older children and people over 65 should start with a low dose and increase as needed.

CONTINUED

The 50 Most Effective Herbs

Red Raspberry
Rubus idaeus

The berry of this biennial bush is commonly used in desserts, but herbalists value the leaves. These have high concentrations of tannin, a chemical that herbalists believe is effective in treating diarrhoea, nausea, vomiting and morning sickness in pregnancy. It is also thought that tannin, an astringent substance, helps prevent miscarriages and, during labour, checks haemorrhaging, strengthens contractions and reduces labour pains; you should not, however, use red raspberry for this purpose at home. Red raspberry leaves are included in several over-the-counter herbal pregnancy formulas. The herb is also used as a gargle for sore throats.

■ TARGET AILMENTS
Take internally for morning sickness, threatened miscarriage, problems during labour, diarrhoea, mouth ulcers, bleeding gums.

PREPARATIONS
Over the counter: Available as dried leaves or berries and as tincture.
At home:
Infusion: Use 1 to 2 tsp dried leaves or berries per 8 fl oz (235 ml) of boiling water. Steep for 10 to 15 minutes. Drink cold and as desired. During pregnancy, steep ½ oz (15 g) dried leaves with 16 fl oz (475 ml) boiling water for 3–5 minutes and drink this amount, warm, each day. For children, dilute with water.

SIDE EFFECTS
Not serious: May cause stomach upset or diarrhoea if you exceed the recommended dose.

SPECIAL INFORMATION
- Pregnant women should take red raspberry only under the supervision of a doctor.
- Animal tests suggest that red raspberry may reduce levels of glucose and so may help diabetes.

Rosemary
Rosmarinus officinalis

Herbalists believe rosemary leaves stimulate the circulatory and nervous systems and are an antidepressant. The leaves are thought to contain anti-spasmodic chemicals that relax the smooth muscle lining of the digestive tract and also are used to treat muscle pain. Rosemary has antibacterial and antifungal properties.

■ TARGET AILMENTS
Take internally for indigestion, upper respiratory tract infections that require a decongestant, tension, muscle pain, sprains, rheumatism, neuralgia.
Apply externally, as an antiseptic, for skin infections.

PREPARATIONS
Over the counter: Available as dried bulk, tincture and two types of oil, one for internal use and the other for external application.
At home:
Tea: Use 1 tsp crushed leaves per 8 fl oz (235 ml) of boiling water. Steep 15 minutes. To settle the stomach or clear a stuffy nose, drink 3 times this amount a day. For children younger than 2, dilute with water.

SIDE EFFECTS
Not serious: Rosemary oil for internal use may cause mild stomach, kidney, and intestinal irritation, even in small doses. If you experience any of these discomforts, consult your doctor.
Serious: Rosemary oil, taken internally in large amounts, can be poisonous. Keep to the prescribed dosage.

SPECIAL INFORMATION
WARNING: Do not confuse rosemary oil for internal use with that for external use.. Never ingest the latter.
- Do not use if you are pregnant.

Saw Palmetto
Serenoa repens

An extract made from the berries of this shrub is used to treat and strengthen the male reproductive system. It is particularly recommended for benign prostatic hyperplasia, or enlargement of the prostate gland. Common among men over 50, the condition is thought to be caused by an accumulation of a testosterone derivative called dihydrotestosterone, which saw palmetto appears to block the production of. The herb has also been used as an expectorant, diuretic, tonic, antiseptic, sedative and digestive aid.

■ TARGET AILMENTS
Take internally for benign prostatic hyperplasia; nasal congestion; asthma and bronchitis; coughs due to colds; sore throats; sinus ailments.

PREPARATIONS
Over the counter: Available as fresh or dried berries and in powder or capsule form. Gel capsules are preferable to tea or tincture.
At home:
Infusion: Steep ½ to 1 tsp fresh berries per 8 fl oz (235 ml) of boiling water for 10 minutes. Drink 6 fl oz (180 ml), two or three times a day.
Decoction: Add ½ to 1 tsp dried berries to 8 fl oz (235 ml) water, bring to a boil, and simmer for 5 minutes. Drink three times daily.
Tincture: Drink 15 to 60 drops in water two or three times daily.

SIDE EFFECTS
None expected.

SPECIAL INFORMATION
WARNING: Do not substitute saw palmetto for medical treatment. Because the symptoms of prostate enlargement and prostate cancer are similar, men should see a doctor when they have symptoms such as urine retention, dribbling and passage of blood in the urine.

The 50 Most Effective Herbs

Skullcap

Scutellaria lateriflora

Skullcap's leaves and blue flowers are used in many over-the-counter herbal sleep remedies. Some researchers report that skullcap calms the nervous system. Chinese medicine physicians use it to treat hepatitis. In the West, however, skullcap is considered controversial and even useless by many medical authorities, at least in part because of its early—and unearned—reputation for curing rabies, for which it garnered the now archaic name of mad dog weed. Its current name comes from a caplike appendage on the upper lip of the flower.

■ TARGET AILMENTS
Take internally for nervous tension; headaches, muscle aches, and symptoms of PMS aggravated or caused by stress; insomnia; convulsions; drug or alcohol withdrawal.

PREPARATIONS
Over the counter: Available as prepared tea, tincture, dried leaves or capsules.
At home:
Tea: Pour 8 fl oz (235 ml) boiling water over 2 tsp dried leaves and steep for 10 to 15 minutes; drink this amount up to three times daily.
Tincture: Take ½ to 1 tsp per 8 fl oz (235 ml) warm water.

SIDE EFFECTS
Not serious: Stomach upset or diarrhoea. Reduce intake or stop using.

SPECIAL INFORMATION
WARNING: Skullcap may cause drowsiness. Do not operate a car or heavy machinery after taking it.
WARNING: Taking large amounts of the tincture may cause confusion, giddiness, twitching and possibly convulsions.
Skullcap in medicinal amounts should be used only under professional supervision.

St John's Wort

Hypericum perforatum

For centuries herbalists have used the blood red flowers of St John's wort to heal wounds and treat depression.

■ TARGET AILMENTS
Use externally for wounds (cuts, abrasions, burns); scar tissue.
Take internally in consultation with a herbalist or a doctor for depression.

PREPARATIONS
Over the counter: Available as dried leaves and flowers, tincture, extract, oil, ointment, capsules and prepared tea.
At home:
Tea: Add 1 to 2 tsp dried herb to 8 fl oz (235 ml) boiling water; steep for 15 minutes. Drink up to 3 times this amount a day.
Oil: Soak the flowers in almond or olive oil until the oil turns bright red.
Ointment: Use a commercial preparation, or warm the leaves in hot petroleum jelly or a mixture of beeswax and almond oil.
Fresh: Apply crushed leaves and flowers to cleansed wounds.
Tincture: Add ¼ to 1 tsp to an 8 fl oz (235 ml) water and drink daily.

SIDE EFFECTS
Serious: High blood pressure, headaches, stiff neck, nausea, and vomiting. Can exacerbate sunburn in the fair-skinned.

SPECIAL INFORMATION
Consult a doctor or a herbalist before using St John's wort.

POSSIBLE INTERACTIONS
WARNING: Avoid the amino acids tryptophan and tyrosine; amphetamines; asthma inhalants; beer, coffee, wine; chocolate, fava beans, salami, smoked or pickled foods and yoghurt; cold or hay fever medicines; diet pills; narcotics; nasal decongestants.

Usnea

Usnea spp.

Usnea, or larch moss, refers to a group of lichens, plants made up of algae and fungi that grow together interdependently. Usnea is found hanging from the larch and many other trees in the Northern Hemisphere. The active ingredient, usnic acid, seems to have an antibiotic effect against the Gram-positive class of bacteria, which includes Streptococcus. It may also be effective against some fungi and protozoans. Usnea is believed to work by disrupting the cell metabolism of bacteria and other simple organisms, though it does not damage human cells. Herbalists consider it an immune system stimulant and a muscle relaxant.

■ TARGET AILMENTS
Take internally for colds, influenza, sore throats, respiratory infections; gastrointestinal irritations.
Apply externally for skin ulcers and fungal infections such as athlete's foot; use as a douche for vaginal infections and urinary tract infections such as urethritis or cystitis.

PREPARATIONS
Over the counter: Available in bulk, powder or tincture.
At home:
Tea: Steep 2–3 tsp dried lichen or 1–2 tsp powder in 8 fl oz (235 ml) boiling water. Take three times daily.

SIDE EFFECTS
Not serious: If digestive disorders arise, reduce dosage. Call your doctor if these symptoms persist.

SPECIAL INFORMATION
WARNING: Pregnant women should avoid using this herb because it may stimulate uterine contractions.
Dilute tincture before ingesting; high concentrations may cause digestive problems.
Do not use for more than three consecutive weeks.

CONTINUED

The 50 Most Effective Herbs

Uva Ursi

Arctostaphylos uva-ursi

Uva ursi, prescribed by herbalists for urinary problems, is also used to treat minor wounds. Its leaves contain arbutin, which is converted in the urinary tract to the antiseptic hydroquinone.

■ **TARGET AILMENTS**

Take internally for mild urinary tract infections, such as urethritis and cystitis; high blood pressure; menstrual bloating.

Apply externally for skin problems such as cuts and abrasions.

PREPARATIONS

Over the counter: Available as dried leaves; as a tincture; and as a tea, alone or in combination with other ingredients.

At home:

Tea: Simmer for 5 to 10 minutes; let stand for 12 to 24 hours. To counteract the effect of the tannin content, add peppermint or chamomile. Drink 24 fl oz (700 ml) a day.

Compress: Make a tea; strain; soak a pad in the tea and apply.

SIDE EFFECTS

Not serious: Taking uva ursi may produce dark green urine; this is harmless. The herb's high tannin content may cause stomach upset.

Serious: A 1949 study involving very high doses of hydroquinone reported tinnitus, nausea and convulsions. Prescribed doses of the whole herb are considered safe; in case of side effects, discontinue taking until you contact your doctor.

SPECIAL INFORMATION

➤ Uva ursi works only in an alkaline environment; avoid acidic foods and vitamin C when taking.

➤ Because hydroquinone is toxic in high doses, use uva ursi only in recommended amounts.

➤ Do not use if you are pregnant; it may stimulate uterine contractions.

Valerian

Valeriana officinalis

Valerian root has been used for more than a thousand years for its calming qualities, and recent research has confirmed its efficacy and safety as a mild tranquillizer and sleep aid. Valerian hastens the onset of sleep, improves sleep quality, and reduces night-time awakenings. Unlike barbiturates or benzodiazepines, prescribed amounts leave no morning grogginess and do not interfere with the vivid dreaming sleep known as REM sleep. It is not habit forming and produces no withdrawal symptoms when discontinued.

■ **TARGET AILMENTS**

Take internally for insomnia, anxiety, nervousness, headache, intestinal pains, menstrual cramps.

PREPARATIONS

Over the counter: Available dried or as capsules, tincture, and teas.

At home:

Tea: Steep 2 tsp dried, chopped root in 8 fl oz (235 ml) boiling water. Let stand 8 to 12 hours. Drink this before bed.

SIDE EFFECTS

Not serious: A mild headache or upset stomach may develop. Reduce dosage. Tell your doctor if it persists.

Serious: More severe headache, restlessness, nausea, morning grogginess or blurred vision may be caused by using too much valerian. Contact your doctor, who will probably tell you to take less or to stop using the herb.

SPECIAL INFORMATION

➤ Do not take valerian with conventional tranquillizers or sedatives, because of possible additive effects.

➤ Paradoxically, valerian may produce excitability in some people.

➤ Be careful about driving until you know how the herb affects you.

Yarrow

Achillea millefolium

Yarrow has been used to heal wounds since ancient times. Modern investigation has revealed many chemicals in this herb that have pain-relieving and anti-inflammatory effects. The leaves, stems and flower tops contain more than 10 active ingredients, including salicylic acid, menthol and camphor. Two major constituents, achilletin and achilleine, are thought to help blood coagulate, while thujone (also found in chamomile) has mild sedative properties. Because yarrow may have diuretic properties, it is sometimes used to treat menstrual bloating and high blood pressure. The somewhat bitter taste of yarrow tea can be relieved by adding sweeteners. A naturalized perennial from Eurasia, yarrow is widely planted in flower and herb gardens.

■ **TARGET AILMENTS**

Take internally for fever, digestive disorders, menstrual cramps, anxiety, insomnia, high blood pressure.

Apply externally for minor wounds, bleeding. Use as a douche for vaginal irritations.

PREPARATIONS

Over the counter: Available as dried herb or tea.

At home:

Tea: Steep 1 to 2 tsp dried herb in 8 fl oz (235 ml) boiling water for 10 to 15 minutes. Drink up to 3 cups a day.

SIDE EFFECTS

Not serious: Yarrow may produce a rash or diarrhoea. Stop using the herb and consult your doctor.

SPECIAL INFORMATION

➤ If you are allergic to ragweed, you may develop a rash from ingesting yarrow.

■

$\mathcal{H}$omoeopathy

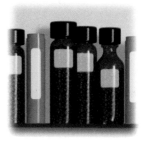

H omoeopathy is a method of healing based on the idea that like cures like; that is, that substances causing specific symptoms in a healthy person can cure these symptoms in someone who is sick. Also called the law of similars, this principle gives homoeopathy its name: 'homoeo' meaning similar, 'pathy' meaning disease. The remedies are prepared from plant, mineral and animal extracts that are highly diluted in a specific way that makes toxicity impossible and, paradoxically, increases their potential to cure.

 Homoeopathic treatment, in its principles and procedures, is unlike any other system of medicinal care. Although there are a few conventional therapies, such as allergy desensitization and immunization, which involve the use of 'similars' to some degree, modern medicine relies almost exclusively on counteracting substances; laxatives, for example, are medications that work to counteract constipation.

Target Ailments

- Allergies
- Arthritis
- Asthma
- Athletic Injuries
- Bladder Infections
- Chronic Fatigue Syndrome
- Common Cold
- Diarrhoea
- Earache
- Fever and Chills
- Flu
- Food Poisoning
- Haemorrhoids
- Hay Fever
- Headache
- Insomnia
- Menstrual Problems
- Motion Sickness
- Pneumonia
- Premenstrual Syndrome
- Sore Throat

Origins

Modern homoeopathy was founded in the 1790s by a German doctor named Samuel Hahnemann. Unhappy with existing medical techniques, Hahnemann experimented with small doses of substances known to cure specific diseases. Just as he had suspected, when given to healthy people these substances induced symptoms of the very diseases they were used to treat. In time, Hahnemann developed a method of preparing remedies by diluting small quantities of herbs, minerals and animal extracts in a water-alcohol solution. The results convinced him that using increasingly smaller amounts of a substance in dilution not only eliminated unwanted side effects but actually boosted the remedy's potency. To unlock these curative powers, though, the solution had to be shaken vigorously. He called his method of preparing remedies potentizing, believing that shaking, or 'succussing', the substances released their stores of vital energy.

Hahnemann was not the first to theorize that cures could be fashioned from the causes of disease. In the fifth century BC, the Greek physician Hippocrates described a system of healing by 'similars'; this notion of fighting illness with like substances contrasted with the more orthodox practice of healing by 'contraries', or antidotes. Over time, medical practitioners came to rely almost exclusively on contraries, deriving treatments from substances that reverse or work against the actions of particular diseases. Yet the principle of similars persisted in folk medicine for hundreds of years, providing Hahnemann with the groundwork for his revolutionary methods.

CONTINUED

Homoeopathy

Testing the Remedies

Most homoeopathic remedies have undergone 'provings', or medical trials in which healthy individuals are given doses of undiluted or slightly diluted substances that are known to cause illnesses. During each test, researchers note the subjects' mental, emotional and physical changes, which together paint a full picture of the symptoms brought on by a given substance. Responses have been recorded over the years in the materia medica, a master reference collection that gives homoeopaths a basis for deciding which remedy is best suited for a patient with a particular set of symptoms.

What It's Good For

Used for a wide range of conditions, homoeopathy is especially effective for noncritical ailments and for those that do not involve severe structural damage or organ destruction. It is also appropriate for diseases for which no effective conventional treatment is available, such as viral illnesses and multiple sclerosis; for ailments that require continuous use of drugs (allergies, arthritis and digestive problems, for example); and for behavioural and emotional disorders.

Although not every remedy has undergone conventional double-blind drug testing, clinical trials have shown a positive effect for a number of conditions, including hay fever, flu, acute childhood diarrhoea, asthma, rheumatoid arthritis, and pain, as well as cardiovascular, respiratory and gastrointestinal diseases. Further research is being conducted in a number of countries.

Preparations/Techniques

Remedies come in a variety of forms, including tablets, powders, wafers and liquids in an alcohol base. Recently, over-the-counter combination remedies have become available for common ailments. These products, labelled according to the name of the ailment, allow self-treatment of such minor conditions as insomnia, flu, sore throat and headache.

The specific dilution of a remedy is the ratio of active substance to inactive base. Ratios containing an x indicate that the remedy consists of 1 part mother tincture (concentrated extract) mixed with 9 parts alcohol base; ratios containing a c consist of 1 part mother tincture and 99 parts base. Further dilutions are represented by a number preceding the x or c. For example, a remedy labelled 30c has first been mixed 1 part to 99; then, 1 part of the resulting mixture is diluted again with 99 parts of the base, and this process is repeated for a total of 30 times. Modern over-the-counter remedies usually have dilution ratios ranging from 1x to 30c; remedies restricted to professional use generally range from 200c to 1,000,000c.

Homoeopathy

When taking homoeopathic remedies in tablet form, be careful not to touch them. Instead, pour the tablets into the bottle cap, then tip them directly on to or under your tongue. If you spill any tablets, throw them away. Practitioners recommend that the mouth be clean of flavours 15 minutes before and after taking a remedy. Avoid strong flavours and aromas—such as mint, camphor, coffee and heavily scented perfumes—for the duration of the treatment.

Visiting a Professional

For chronic problems, most practitioners practice 'constitutional' homoeopathy, which is based on the idea that the patient's constitution must be considered along with the disease itself. Acute, or short-term, conditions are usually treated with remedies specific to the illness. Typically, the practitioner takes an extensive medical history of the patient, notes the physical and psychological symptoms, then prescribes a single remedy. If this prescription does not have the desired effect, the homoeopath performs another analysis and gives a second prescription. Symptom analysis is the key to success; consequently, two patients suffering from the same disorder but displaying different symptoms may receive different prescriptions.

If the correct remedy has been prescribed, healing may begin immediately or within a few days or weeks. When it does, stop taking the remedy, and start again only if your symptoms return. In some cases a prescription will cause what's known as an aggravation, or a temporary worsening of your symptoms. This is usually an indication that the remedy is going to work. Stop taking it and wait for the positive effect.

Well-being

Homoeopathic practitioners often provide constitutional treatments—regimens based on personal and family medical histories—to patients who are not sick but want to maintain or improve their general health.

What the Critics Say

Critics argue that some homoeopathic remedies are so diluted they no longer contain even a single molecule of the original healing substance. Many homoeopathic remedies have been proved effective in clinical trials, but opponents attribute any therapeutic success to the placebo effect. The idea that a substance can cure by releasing energy, say sceptics, puts homoeopathy in the realm of metaphysics. ■

FOR MORE INFO
Following is a list of organizations you can contact to learn more about homoeopathy:

British Homoeopathic Association
27a Devonshire Street
London W1N 1RJ
020 7935 2163

United Kingdom Homoeopathic Medical Association
6 Livingstone Road
Gravesend
Kent DA12 5DZ
01474 560336

Society of Homoeopaths
2 Artizan Road
Northampton NN1 4HU
01604 621400
fax: 01604 622622
email: societyofhomoeopaths
@btinternet.com

The 24 Most Effective Homoeopathic Remedies

Aconite · *Aconitum napellus*

Aconite grows throughout the mountainous regions of Europe, Russia and central Asia, producing clusters of bluish violet flowers that hang from the stem like monks' cowls, giving the plant its common name, monkshood. Highly toxic, aconite was the preferred poison of the ancient Greeks. Administered in very small doses, it produces mental and physical restlessness and tissue inflammation. Homoeopaths prescribe *Aconite* for those patients whose symptoms resemble the effects of the poison—who seem distressed or fearful and complain of thirst and unbearable aches and pains that accompany their illnesses.

For homoeopathic use, the whole plant—except the root, which is the most poisonous part—is gathered while in full bloom and pounded to a pulp. Juice is pressed from the pulp and mixed with alcohol, then diluted to non-toxic levels.

TARGET AILMENTS

Angina, arrhythmia, anxiety induced by sudden shock, arthritis, asthma, bronchitis, colds and flu, croup, fevers with rapid onset and chills that may be accompanied by restlessness or thirst, eye inflammations with burning pain and sensitivity to light, laryngitis, sore throat, middle ear infections, toothaches with a sensitivity to cold water.

Allium cepa · *Allium cepa*

Cultivated worldwide, *Allium cepa*, otherwise known as red onion, has been used in folk medicine for centuries. This common garden vegetable has been applied to the skin in poultices for acne, arthritis and congestion, and used internally to clear worms from the intestines. Modern-day herbalists find onion useful for treating conditions as varied as earaches, haemorrhoids and high blood pressure. Homoeopathic practitioners consider *Allium cepa* a remedy for conditions that are accompanied by the same symptoms as those brought on by exposure to red onions—watering eyes and a burning, runny nose.

For the homoeopathic preparation, red onions are harvested in midsummer. The bulbs are pounded to a pulp and then mixed with water and alcohol through several stages of extreme dilution.

TARGET AILMENTS

Colds with sinus congestion that shifts from side to side in the head; coughs that cause a ripping, tearing pain in the throat; watery and inflamed eyes, hay fever; neuralgic pains; earaches.

Apis · *Apis mellifica*

The medicinal value of *Apis*, the scientific name for the honeybee, may date back to ancient Egypt, where bees were a symbol of power, wealth and health. Egyptian doctors revered honey over all other healing substances, and extensive methods of beekeeping were already in practice in 4000 BC. It is not the honey but the bee itself, however, that is used in homoeopathic medicine.

This remedy is made from the body of the honeybee; it is used to treat those patients whose ailments are accompanied by symptoms similar to the results of a bee sting, such as redness and swelling, and also patients who express behaviour considered bee-like, such as restlessness or irritability. To prepare this remedy, the entire live honeybee is crushed and highly diluted by mixing it into a water-and-alcohol base.

TARGET AILMENTS

Bites and stings, especially those that burn, itch or swell; conjunctivitis; oedema (accumulation of fluids in body tissues) and conditions of general swelling such as nettle rash and food allergies; headaches that include sudden, stabbing pains; red, swollen joints; mumps.

The 24 Most Effective Homoeopathic Remedies

Arsenicum album · *Arsenicum album*

This remedy, also called *Ars alb* by homoeopathic practitioners, is an extremely dilute form of arsenic, a metallic poison derived from the chemical element of the same name. Weak preparations of arsenic have had a history of medicinal use; but slow accumulation of the element in body tissues can cause chronic poisoning, leading to gastrointestinal disorders, nausea, dehydration and even paralysis and death. In step with the homoeopathic theory that like cures like, *Ars alb* is preferred by practitioners to treat patients with various digestive complaints that are accompanied by signs of dehydration and burning pains, the same symptoms that are induced by arsenic.

In its homoeopathic form, arsenic is separated from other metals such as iron, cobalt and nickel by baking at high temperatures. The extracted powder is then finely ground and weakened by mixing successively greater amounts of lactose (milk sugar) with the poison.

TARGET AILMENTS

Angina; anxiety disorders and panic attacks; asthma; hay fever; burns that form blisters; chronic skin problems; high fevers accompanied by chills; recurrent headaches; dry, hacking coughs; colds accompanied by excessive, watery nasal discharge and frequent sneezing; colitis, indigestion, food poisoning, Crohn's disease; influenza; insomnia; exhaustion from an illness coupled with restlessness.

Belladonna · *Belladonna*

Belladonna, a highly toxic plant also known as deadly nightshade, grows wild across Europe, producing yellow flowers in July and dark red berries in late summer. Its name, meaning 'beautiful woman' in Italian, dates from the Renaissance, when ladies of Italy dilated their pupils with belladonna eye drops for a doe-eyed appearance. Belladonna poisoning brings on a range of symptoms, including a dry mouth and hot, flushed skin, nausea, convulsive movements and delirium. Homoeopathic practitioners prescribe *Belladonna* for illnesses that are accompanied by these same symptoms. All parts of the belladonna plant are gathered for use in the homoeopathic remedy. The plant is crushed and pressed, and the extracted juice is mixed with alcohol in an extremely dilute preparation.

TARGET AILMENTS

Common cold, flu, sore throat, painful earache, high fever with chills but with no thirst, acute inflammatory arthritis, acute bursitis, gallstones, colic, measles, mumps, acute diverticulitis, neuralgia, sunstroke, acutely inflamed varicose veins, painful toothache, painful menstrual periods, teething pains, breast-feeding complications.

Bryonia · *Bryonia alba*

Bryonia, or wild hops, is a creeping vine commonly found along hedgerows and in forests across southern Europe. Its medicinal value was known to the Greeks, who used the root as a purgative and may have given the plant its name, derived from *bryo*, meaning 'to thrust or sprout', a reference to how quickly the vine grows. Accidental ingestion of the root can cause tissue inflammation, severe vomiting and diarrhoea violent enough to cause death. Homoeopaths prescribe their dilute solutions of *Bryonia* for illnesses that are accompanied by similar symptoms. The homoeopathic remedy is prepared from the root, which is harvested in early spring. An extract pressed from the root pulp is mixed with alcohol into an extremely dilute solution.

TARGET AILMENTS

Arthritis with sharp, sticking pains; backaches centred in the small of the back; bursitis; colds accompanied by chest congestion; painful coughs; sore throat with pain upon swallowing; influenza; severe headaches worsened by light, sound or motion; dizziness; nausea, vomiting, constipation, gastritis, acute diverticulitis, stomach flu; inflammation during breast-feeding.

CONTINUED

The 24 Most Effective Homoeopathic Remedies

Calcarea carbonica • *Calcarea carbonica*

Calcarea carbonica, or calcium carbonate, is a source of calcium, one of the most abundant natural elements in the human body. Essential to cell structure and bone strength, calcium comes from many materials, including chalk, coral and limestone. Perhaps as a reflection of its body-building properties, *Calcarea carbonica*, also called *Calc carb*, is used by homoeopaths for conditions that are accompanied by symptoms of exhaustion, depression, and anxiety. Calcium carbonate prepared for homoeopathic use is ground from oyster shells and used at full strength.

TARGET AILMENTS

Lower-back pain, broken bones, sprains, muscle cramps, constipation, chronic ear infections, eye inflammations, headaches, insomnia, eczema, allergies, teething problems, gastritis, gallstones, childhood diarrhoea, menstrual problems, asthma, palpitations, arthritis.

Cantharis • *Cantharis*

Popularly known as Spanish fly, *Cantharis* is actually a beetle found in southern France and Spain. It produces an irritant so caustic that the skin will blister if exposed to it.

Cantharis has had a long career in medicine and has been used for all manner of disorders. In high concentrations the irritant can be toxic, prompting abdominal cramps and burning pains in the throat and stomach, vomiting of blood, diarrhoea, kidney damage, convulsions, coma and death. Homoeopaths prescribe *Cantharis* for patients whose ailments are coupled with symptoms like those of cantharis poisoning.

According to homoeopathic tradition, the beetles are collected at daybreak, when they are still sluggish from the cool of the night, and heated in the steam of boiling vinegar until dead. The beetles are then crushed and mixed with successively greater amounts of milk sugar, a pharmaceutical process called trituration. The resulting powder is highly dilute.

TARGET AILMENTS

Bladder infections or cystitis, with a constant desire to urinate accompanied by blood and pain during urination; sunburns, scalds and blistering second-degree burns.

Chamomilla • *Chamomilla*

Chamomilla is made from the flowering German chamomile plant common in Europe. The whole plant is crushed, and its juices are mixed with equal parts of alcohol, then succussed. In homoeopathy *Chamomilla* is considered to work best for people who are extremely sensitive to pain, irritable, impatient and implacable. *Chamomilla* patients sweat easily and are sensitive to wind and chills. *Chamomilla* is most often given to children who work themselves into violent temper tantrums.

TARGET AILMENTS

Irritability; toothaches aggravated by cold air and warm food; painful menstrual periods with severe cramping and a feeling of anger or restlessness; extremely painful earaches; teething pain, especially if the child is irritable; difficulty getting to sleep.

The 24 Most Effective Homoeopathic Remedies

Ferrum phosphoricum • *Ferrum phosphoricum*

Ferrum phosphoricum, also called *Ferrum phos* or iron phosphate, is a mineral compound of iron and phosphorus. Both elements are present in the body independently; iron aids the exchange of oxygen in the blood, and phosphorus contributes to bone and muscle health. *Ferrum phos* is derived from mixing solutions of iron sulphate, phosphate and sodium acetate. The resulting iron phosphate is ground with large quantities of lactose (milk sugar) to render it non-toxic. Homoeopathic practitioners consider *Ferrum phos* good for patients who suffer from conditions accompanied by low energy and anaemia.

TARGET AILMENTS

Tickling, hacking coughs with chest pain, headaches, fevers that begin slowly, ear infections, incontinence, rheumatic joints, early menstrual periods accompanied by headaches, anaemia, fatigue, nosebleeds, sore throat, vomiting, diarrhoea, palpitations.

Hepar sulphuris • *Hepar sulphuris calcareum*

The flaky inner layer of oyster shells provides the calcium used in this homoeopathic remedy, also called *Hepar sulph* and commonly known as calcium sulphide. Once an antidote for mercury poisoning, *Hepar sulphuris* is now used by homoeopaths to treat patients with conditions that tend to be infected, often producing pus. These disorders are accompanied by symptoms that include mental and physical hypersensitivity and an intolerance of pain and cold.

Finely ground oyster shell and sulphur are mixed together and then heated in an airtight container. The resulting powder is dissolved in hot hydrochloric acid, then combined with lactose (milk sugar) in a pharmaceutical process of dilution called trituration.

TARGET AILMENTS

Abscesses that are swollen and painful but have not yet opened; colds, sore throat and earache; inflamed cuts and wounds that may be taking longer than normal to heal; aching joints; fits of coughing with chest pain, hoarseness, asthma, emphysema, croup; genital herpes; constipation.

Hypericum • *Hypericum perforatum*

Also known as St John's wort, hypericum grows in woodlands across Europe, Asia and North America, blooming with a profusion of yellow flowers from June to September. The flowers, if bruised, bleed a reddish juice. The dark green leaves of the plant are dotted with oil-producing pores. According to ancient healing wisdom, because hypericum seemed to resemble skin, with its pores and its simulation of bleeding on injury, it was considered ideal for all manner of flesh wounds. (*See St John's Wort, page 75.*) In homoeopathy *Hypericum* is often prescribed for bodily injuries, among other conditions, but it is selected for the soothing effect it is said to have on injured nerves rather than for any traditional reason.

For homoeopathic use the entire plant is harvested in summer, when its yellow flowers are in full bloom. It is pounded to a pulp and soaked in an alcohol solution before being weakened to the desired potencies through a vigorous dilution process.

TARGET AILMENTS

Backaches centred along the lower spine that may include shooting pains; bites and stings from animals and insects, especially when they have become inflamed or include nerve damage; cuts and wounds in nerve-rich parts of the body, such as the fingers and lips, caused by accidents or surgery.

CONTINUED

The 24 Most Effective Homoeopathic Remedies

Ignatia • *Ignatia amara*

The beans of this plant, sometimes called St Ignatius bean, are in fact seeds from the fruit of a small tree native to China and the Philippines. Spanish missionaries in the Philippines were introduced to the seeds by the locals, who wore them as amulets to ward off disease. Small doses of the seed can produce mild but unpleasant symptoms of poisoning, including increased salivation, pounding headache, cramps, giddiness, twitching and trembling; large doses can be fatal. Homoeopaths may prescribe *Ignatia*, a dilute solution of the seed, for ailments that include symptoms like those associated with mild poisoning.

For the homoeopathic preparation, seeds are collected and ground to a powder, then mixed with alcohol. When the powder is saturated, the mixture is strained and diluted until it becomes a non-toxic substance.

TARGET AILMENTS

Anxiety; dry, tickling coughs; a sore throat that feels like there is a lump in it; painful tension headaches; indigestion; insomnia; irritable bowel syndrome; painful haemorrhoids; effects of grief, shock or disappointment, or depression where the patient tends to sigh frequently.

Ipecac • *Ipecacuanha*

The *Ipecacuanha* shrub, native to Central and South America, was named by Portuguese colonists, who called it 'roadside sick-making plant' in recognition of its ability to induce vomiting. Varying dosages of its root can produce a variety of symptoms, including mild appetite stimulation, sweating, expectoration, vomiting, gastritis, inflammation of the lungs, and cardiac failure. Other health disorders can display symptoms similar to those of mild ipecac poisoning, and it is these symptoms that homoeopathic practitioners hope to counteract when they prescribe *Ipecac*.

The homoeopathic remedy is made from the root, the most potent part. The root is dried and then ground into a coarse powder, which is diluted either in milk sugar to be used as a dry substance or in a water-and-alcohol base. Both preparations are weakened to a non-toxic level.

TARGET AILMENTS

Persistent nausea, vomiting, motion sickness; menstrual problems; asthma; dry, irritating cough accompanied by wheezing; diarrhoea; flu with nausea; colic; gastroenteritis.

Kali bichromicum • *Kali bichromicum*

Kali bichromicum is often called potassium bichromate; it is a chemical compound that may be acquired from chromium iron ore or by processing potassium chromate with one of a number of strong acids. A highly corrosive substance, it is used primarily in textile dyeing, in the staining of wood, and as a component in electric batteries. It is also a very powerful poison. Homoeopathic practitioners believe *Kali bichromicum* works best for conditions that are accompanied by the symptom of pain in a distinct spot, where the ache is easily located with a fingertip.

For homoeopathic use this caustic chemical, also called *Kali bi*, is diluted to non-toxic levels with large amounts of milk sugar, a pharmaceutical process called trituration.

TARGET AILMENTS

Acute bronchitis, colds in which there is a thick mucus discharge and a heavy cough that produces pain in the chest, croup, sinusitis and resulting headaches, indigestion, pains in the joints.

The 24 Most Effective Homoeopathic Remedies

Lycopodium • *Lycopodium clavatum*

Lycopodium, also known as club moss, grows in pastures and woodlands throughout Britain, northern Europe and North America. Its spores contain a highly flammable pollen that was once used in fireworks and other pyrotechnics. Powder made from its ground-up spores has been used for internal complaints such as diarrhoea and dysentery since the 17th century. Homoeopaths use dilute doses of *Lycopodium* for complaints that are accompanied by symptoms of digestive upset, ailments that seem to develop on the right side of the body, a strong desire for sweets, anxiety and symptoms that worsen in the early evening. To create the homoeopathic remedy, pollen is extracted from the spores and diluted with milk sugar.

TARGET AILMENTS

Backache with stiffness and soreness in the lower back, bedwetting, colds with stuffy nose, constipation, coughs with mucus, cystitis, headache with throbbing pain, gout, indigestion accompanied by abdominal cramps, wind, heartburn, joint pain, sciatica, right-sided sore throat, eczema.

Mercurius vivus • *Mercurius vivus*

One of the metallic chemical elements, mercury, also called quicksilver, was known in ancient Chinese and Hindu civilizations and has had a long history of medicinal use. Ingesting certain mercury compounds can cause increased perspiration and salivation; and so in ancient medicine mercury was used, along with bloodletting and purging, as a means of ridding the body of impurities. Undilute mercury is toxic, however, and severe symptoms of mercury poisoning may include nausea, inflammation of the digestive tract and kidney failure.

Homoeopathic practitioners prescribe *Merc viv*, as the homoeopathic preparation of mercury is sometimes called, for conditions accompanied by symptoms of shaking, hot and cold sweats, and restlessness. *Merc viv* is made from the chemical element mercury by dilution with large quantities of milk sugar.

TARGET AILMENTS

Abscesses, especially dental or glandular; backache with burning, shooting pains in the lower back; chicken pox; colds with an exceptionally runny nose and pain in the nostrils; cystitis with slow urination; painful diarrhoea; influenza; earache with discharge of pus; eye inflammation; indigestion; mouth ulcers; burning sore throat; toothache with increased salivation.

Natrum muriaticum • *Natrum muriaticum*

Natrum muriaticum is simply salt, or sodium chloride, a substance present in the natural world in quantities greater than any other except water. Essential to life and health, salt has been valued in human commerce throughout history. Roman soldiers were given a stipend, called a salarium, which they used to buy salt; from this we get the word *salary*. Homoeopaths prescribe dilute solutions of *Nat mur*, as they call it, for conditions that are coupled with symptoms of extreme thirst, emotional sensitivity and a strong desire for salt.

Nat mur is prepared by adding pure sodium chloride to boiling water. Once the salt has dissolved, the solution is filtered and crystallized by evaporation. The final product is diluted in water to the desired potency.

TARGET AILMENTS

Backaches that are relieved by firm pressure; cold sores, especially in the corners of the mouth; colds with sneezing, watery eyes, and runny nose; constipation; fevers accompanied by weakness and chills; genital herpes; eczema; anaemia; hay fever; migraine headaches; menstrual irregularity; indigestion; depression caused by grief, with a desire to be alone.

CONTINUED

The 24 Most Effective Homoeopathic Remedies

Nux vomica · *Nux vomica*

Nux vomica, also known as poison nut, is a remedy made from the seeds of an evergreen tree indigenous to parts of India, Thailand, China and Australia. The seeds contain strychnine and have a bitter, unpleasant taste. Small doses of the seed stimulate the appetite, while somewhat larger doses decrease the appetite and cause motor dysfunction, including stiffness in the arms and legs and a staggering walk. Toxic doses can cause convulsions and death. *Nux vomica* is prescribed by homoeopaths for ailments that occur from over-indulgence in food, coffee or alcohol, usually accompanied by irritability. To prepare the homoeopathic remedy, poison-nut seeds are ground to a powder and then diluted with milk sugar to the desired potency.

TARGET AILMENTS

Colic and stomach cramps from overeating, colds with sneezing and a stuffy nose, constipation, cystitis, headache with dizziness, fevers with chills, wind and painful wind, hangovers, indigestion, insomnia, irritable bowel syndrome, nausea, menstrual cramps with a heavy flow, sinusitis, stomach flu, vomiting from overeating or eating rich foods.

Phosphorus · *Phosphorus*

The chemical element phosphorus can be found in the cellular fluid of all living tissue. Phosphorus plays a vital role in the activity of the body's cells, most importantly in the transfer of genetic information. Many phosphorus compounds are used commercially in toothpaste, fertilizer and laundry detergent. Phosphorus poisoning causes irritation of the mucous membranes and inflammation of tissue; over time, it can destroy bone. As a homoeopathic remedy, minute doses are prescribed by practitioners for conditions accompanied by symptoms of fatigue and nervousness with a tendency to bleed easily and an unquenchable thirst for cold water. Pure phosphorus is diluted in large quantities of milk sugar to prepare the homoeopathic remedy.

TARGET AILMENTS

Bronchitis, pneumonia, coughs with congestion and burning pains in the chest, visual problems resulting from eyestrain, gastritis, nosebleeds, indigestion accompanied by vomiting or pain, stomach ulcers, kidney infections, nasal polyps, hepatitis, anaemia, haemorrhages, diarrhoea, menstrual problems.

Pulsatilla · *Pulsatilla nigricans*

Common in the meadowlands of northern and central Europe, the pulsatilla, or windflower, contains a caustic substance, and chewing the plant may cause blisters in the mouth and throat. Homoeopaths often prescribe *Pulsatilla* to patients with conditions accompanied by a thick yellow or white discharge. For homoeopathic use the plant is collected when in full bloom and pounded to a pulp. The pulp is steeped in an alcohol-and-water solution and then strained and diluted.

TARGET AILMENTS

Bedwetting, breast infections, chicken pox, coughs, headaches, eye inflammation, fever with chills, hay fever, incontinence, indigestion, aching joints that improve with movement and cold compresses, urethritis in men, late menstrual periods, otitis media, sciatica, sinusitis, varicose veins, depression.

The 24 Most Effective Homoeopathic Remedies

Rhus toxicodendron • *Rhus toxicodendron*

This vine-like shrub, also known as poison ivy, grows throughout North America and is well known for the itchy red rash its oil can cause on the skin. The medicinal history of its leaves and stalk began in the late 18th century, when it was used to treat conditions such as paralysis and rheumatism. The effects of its undilute form can range from a rash to nausea, fever, delirium, swollen glands and ulcers in the oral cavity. For this reason homoeopathic practitioners use *Rhus toxicodendron,* or *Rhus tox,* as it is also called, to treat conditions that may be accompanied by fever, restlessness and swollen glands.

Rhus tox is prepared from plants gathered at night, when the oil is said to be in its most potent state. The leaves and stalks are pounded to a pulp and mixed with alcohol, then strained and diluted.

TARGET AILMENTS

Arthritis with stiffness worse in the morning and better with motion; backache with stiffness along the spine; bursitis; carpal tunnel syndrome; eye inflammation with swelling, itching and stickiness; genital herpes; hamstring injury; influenza with painful joints; headaches; nettle rash that itches and intensifies after scratching; joint and back pains from over-exertion; impetigo; sprains with stiffness; toothaches.

Silica • *Silica*

Silica, also called flint, is a mineral that is present in the human body in only trace amounts but is vital to the development of bones, the flexibility of cartilage and the health of the skin and connective tissues. Many industrial operations rely on silica, including the manufacture of concrete, paper, glass and enamelware. Flint's medicinal use is limited to homoeopathy. Minute doses are prescribed for patients with conditions accompanied by excessive sweating, weakness, and extreme sensitivity to cold. For homoeopathic use silica powder is mixed with sodium carbonate through a pharmaceutical process of dry substance dilution.

TARGET AILMENTS

Athlete's foot, constipation, wounds that have been inflamed by foreign matter, earache with decreased hearing and a stopped-up sensation, fingernails that have white spots and split easily, headaches beginning in the back of the head and spreading forward to the eyes, abscesses, swollen glands in the neck, gum infections, haemorrhoids, breast cysts.

Sulphur • *Sulphur*

The chemical element sulphur is present in all living tissue. It was known to ancient societies, and in the Bible it is called brimstone. Among the various conditions to which it has been applied as a medication for some 2,000 years are skin disorders such as scabies. Commercially, sulphur is used in the production of dyes, fungicides and gunpowder. Homoeopaths may prescribe dilute doses of the remedy *Sulphur* to treat conditions accompanied by irritability, intense itching, burning pains and offensive odours. The homoeopathic remedy is made from pure sulphur powder that is diluted with either milk sugar or a water-and-alcohol solution.

TARGET AILMENTS

Asthma that is worse at night and is accompanied by rattling mucus, cough with chest pain, morning diarrhoea, eye inflammation, bursitis, headaches with burning pain, indigestion, joint pain, anal itching with redness, burning vaginal discharge, eczema with intense itching and burning.

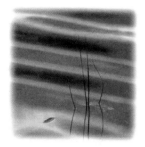

Target Ailments

- Arthritis
- Athletic Injuries
- Bursitis
- Circulatory Problems
- Common Cold
- Fever and Chills
- Haemorrhoids
- Headache
- Indigestion
- Muscle Cramps
- Pain, Chronic
- Rashes and Skin Problems
- Sinusitis
- Stress
- Tendinitis
- Varicose Veins

Hydrotherapy

H ydrotherapy, which literally means water therapy, encompasses a variety of therapeutic uses of water. As either ice, liquid or steam, water may relieve the symptoms of numerous types of infections, acute and chronic pain, circulatory problems and more. External hydrotherapy treatments typically involve applications of hot or cold water (or the alternation of both) to the skin. Internal treatments consist of water taken internally as a cleansing agent.

Treatments range from the homey footbath to sophisticated physical therapy in a hospital pool, and can include wraps, sprays and douches, as well as the use of steam rooms, saunas and hot and cold baths. In general, the aim is to stimulate an immune response or to detoxify the body by changing body temperature.

Origins

Using water as a source of healing is a concept as old as civilization itself. In its modern form, hydrotherapy originated in Germany, where the 19th-century passion for spas and water treatments influenced such healers as the Austrian peasant Vincenz Priessnitz, the founder of hydrotherapy; and Father Sebastian Kneipp, the originator of 'Kneipp's cure', which employed forms of hydrotherapy. By the turn of the century, the term 'water cure' had become a catch-all phrase for many forms of natural healing. Ultimately, hydrotherapy became one of the key treatments of naturopathy *(pages 112-114),* and today, outside the home, it is practised primarily by naturopaths and physical therapists.

What It's Good For

Hydrotherapy has a wide range of applications, but it is particularly useful for treating muscle and joint pain and inflammation, burns and frostbite, sinusitis, fevers, headaches, the upper respiratory tract, indigestion, pelvic pain and stress. In pools and whirlpool baths, hydrotherapy is also used to strengthen limbs after injury. Internal hydrotherapy can ease digestive problems and help detoxify the blood.

Preparations/Techniques

External hydrotherapy relies primarily on the effects of water temperature—hot, neutral, cold or alternating hot and cold—to produce its effects. Hot water soothes and relaxes while stimulating the immune system. Neutral or body-temperature baths are also soothing, particularly for people with stress and insomnia. Cold water discourages inflammation and fever, while the contrast of hot and cold can improve circulation and reduce congestion.

Hydrotherapy

A practitioner might recommend treatments either at a facility with the right kinds of pools and whirlpool tubs, or at home. Some treatments should take place under the watchful eye of a trained doctor or therapist—hyperthermia, for example, which is a fever-inducing therapy for patients fighting viruses and infections. Paraplegics, those suffering from burns and frostbite and anyone with diminished sensation also need to work with therapists if they are being treated in baths.

However, many of the treatments of hydrotherapy can easily be done at home. A simple example is the cold compress. For an inflamed joint or a feverish headache, take a terry cloth flannel, wring it out in ice water and apply it to the afflicted area. As the flannel warms up, chill it down again and repeat.

To improve immune function and for general stimulation, a hydrotherapist might suggest immediately following a hot shower with a cold one. Or if a handheld hose or sprayer is available, you can hook up the sprayer to a tap after a hot shower and spray (or ask a friend to spray) cold water along both sides of the spine.

Hydrotherapists may also recommend adding therapeutic herbs and oils to the bath. Among them could be chamomile to soothe the skin, oatmeal for nettle rash or sunburn, or ginger for relaxation. *(See Herbal Therapies, pages 56-59).*

Well-being

Proponents of hydrotherapy believe that a healthy body maintains a certain internal balance. In order to keep this stability, it must constantly adjust to environmental influences such as heat, cold, food and water, and clothing. Water therapies enhance and reinforce the body's reaction to these external influences, helping it to stay well.

What the Critics Say

Most forms of external hydrotherapy—whirlpool baths, cold compresses and the like—are widely accepted by the medical establishment. Internal hydrotherapy, particularly the use of enemas and colonic irrigation, comes in for more criticism, however. Critics say that such methods have little scientific justification and that they can actually spread infection if not carefully applied. ■

FOR MORE INFO

Following is a list of organizations you can contact to learn more about hydrotherapy:

The UK College of Hydrotherapy
515 Hagley Road
Birmingham B66 4AX
0121 429 9191

The British Naturopathic and Osteopathic Association
Frazer House
6 Netherall Gardens
London NW3 5RR

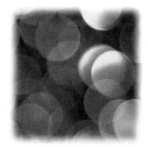

Light Therapy

S imply put, light therapy is the use of light to promote healing. Specific techniques differ primarily in the type of light involved. Full-spectrum light therapy consists of regular exposure to controlled amounts of sunlight or artificial light that contains all wavelengths of light, from infrared to ultraviolet. Bright light therapy involves exposure to non-ultraviolet white light in levels that match the amount of natural sunlight found outdoors shortly after sunrise or before sunset. In cold laser therapy, small beams of low-intensity laser light are applied directly to the skin. Coloured light therapy focuses different coloured lights on the skin.

Target Ailments

- Arthritis
- Carpal Tunnel Syndrome
- Depression
- Headache
- High Blood Pressure
- Insomnia
- Menstrual Problems
- Pain, Chronic
- Premenstrual Syndrome
- Rashes and Skin Problems
- Seasonal Affective Disorder
- Stress
- Tendinitis

The Importance of Light

Recent research indicates that for the body to be healthy, it must receive adequate exposure to the full and balanced spectrum of light found in natural sunlight. Adequate light is especially needed for the regulation of circadian rhythms, the daily internal pacemakers that govern a host of biological functions in humans, from hormone production to patterns of sleeping and waking. In healthy people, these rhythms run in regular cycles, reset each morning by the light of the rising sun. If the rhythms become disturbed for any reason, health problems can result.

Origins

Sunlight has been used for healing throughout history. The ancient Greek physician Hippocrates prescribed sunlight for certain disorders, often sending his patients to recuperate in roofless buildings. During the Middle Ages, red light was a popular treatment for smallpox. The windows of sickrooms were covered with red curtains, and patients were wrapped in red sheets. Doctors started using bright light therapy for seasonal affective disorder and other ailments beginning in the 1980s.

What It's Good For

Full-spectrum light therapy is used to treat various ailments, including high blood pressure, rashes and skin problems, depression, insomnia, PMS, migraines, jaundice in newborns and jet lag. Bright light therapy has been shown to be highly effective in treating seasonal affective disorder (SAD), a form of depression that strikes people during winter, when days are short. Bright light therapy is also used to treat bulimia, irregular menstrual cycles and sleep disorders. Cold laser therapy is used primarily to relieve chronic pain and help heal wounds, but it is also a part of laser acupuncture, a form of acupuncture that addresses a variety of health concerns. Coloured light therapy is used for depression, sleep problems, chronic pain, stress, menstrual problems, arthritis, tendinitis, sore throat, nettle rash and insect bites.

Light Therapy

Preparations/Techniques

Most light therapy can be self-administered, either by spending more time outdoors or by purchasing special therapeutic lights and then following the directions that come with them. Full-spectrum light therapy is accomplished indoors by installing full-spectrum lighting in place of incandescent and fluorescent lighting, which lacks the complete balanced spectrum of sunlight. Bright light therapy requires that you sit near a light box, usually for about 30 minutes, early in the morning from late autumn through early spring. Cold lasers are held over the affected area of the body for specified lengths of time, generally no more than a few minutes. The treatment is then repeated once or twice a day for several days or until the condition improves. Some forms of coloured light therapy also involve directing small beams of light, usually red, over the area of the body that needs healing. Another method involves bathing the body with coloured light from filtered floodlights.

Visiting a Professional

You may find it useful to consult a knowledgeable doctor about applying some forms of light therapy to your particular health concern. Before using bright light therapy for the treatment of SAD, you should see a doctor skilled in the diagnosis and treatment of that illness. Ultraviolet light therapy treatments for dermatitis, psoriasis and other skin problems should be administered only by a professional.

Well-being

People who use light therapy report that it reduces stress and relaxes and rejuvenates the body, thus contributing to an overall feeling of physical and mental well-being. Research has also shown that exposure to full-spectrum and bright light helps promote well-being by keeping the body's biological rhythms synchronized.

What the Critics Say

Although the use of light therapy for the treatment of seasonal affective disorder and skin problems is widely accepted, other forms of light therapy have not undergone rigorous scientific studies. ■

FOR MORE INFO
Following is an organization you can contact to learn more about light therapy:

Outside In (Cambridge) Ltd
21 Scotland Road Estate
Dry Drayton
Cambridge CB3 8AT
01954 211 955
fax: 01954 211 956
email: info@outsidein.co.uk
website: www.outsidein.co.uk

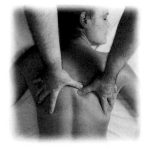

$\mathcal{M}$assage

Target Ailments

- Arthritis
- Asthma
- Athletic Injuries
- Back Problems
- Carpal Tunnel Syndrome
- Chronic Fatigue Syndrome
- Constipation
- Depression
- Headache
- Heartburn
- Immune Problems
- Insomnia
- Irritable Bowel Syndrome
- Multiple Sclerosis
- Muscle Cramps
- Neuralgia
- Pain, Chronic
- Premenstrual Syndrome
- Stomach Ulcers
- Tendinitis
- TMJ Syndrome

$\boxed{M}$ *assage therapy, defined as the systematic manipulation of the soft tissues, relieves sore muscles and promotes relaxation. It is usually performed with various standard hand strokes, but sometimes pressure is applied with other parts of the body, such as the forearm, elbow or foot.*

The general purposes of massage are to reduce tension, improve circulation, aid in the healing of soft-tissue injuries, control pain and promote overall well-being. Massage can gently stretch tissues, increase range of motion and reduce some types of oedema (swelling). It can also help lower blood pressure and heart rate and improve respiration. Researchers believe massage helps the brain make endorphins, chemicals that act as natural pain-killers—which perhaps explains why recipients feel better and more tranquil after a massage.

The Nature of Touch

Touching is, of course, an integral part of massage, and it may play a significant role in massage's therapeutic effects. Studies have found that animals that are touched grow faster and that infants who are not touched develop more slowly, physically and psychologically, than those who are. Touch can convey the therapeutic emotions of caring and concern. Some massage therapists believe that touch can create trust and openness and help release blocked emotions.

Origins

One of the earliest forms of healing, massage was mentioned in Chinese medical texts 4,000 years ago. It has been advocated in Western societies since the Greek physician Hippocrates, in the fourth century BC, referred to a technique called *anatripsis* - literally 'rubbing up'. Massage schools were an integral part of greek gymnasiums and the practice remained popular for the duration of the Roman Empire. Julius Caesar is believed to have had himself pinched all over every day to help treat his neuralgia.

At the beginning of the 19th century, a Swedish gymnastics instructor and fencing master, Pehr Henrik Ling, cured himself of an elbow ailment with percussion strokes (tapping movements). He subsequently developed a method of healing that became known as Swedish massage. This therapy, which was based on the then-emerging science of physiology, came to Britain and the United States in the mid-19th century. Interest dwindled, however, when healthcare took a technological turn in the early 1900s and didn't pick up again until the alternative healthcare movement gained momentum in the 1970s.

Massage

What It's Good For

Massage is recommended for countless injuries and ailments. Well-designed studies have proved the benefits of particular methods of massage to treat pain, nausea, muscle spasm and soft-tissue problems, as well as anxiety, depression, insomnia and emotional stress. Massage helps premature infants gain weight and develop motor skills, and it helps elderly people relax. Researchers believe it also may improve immune system response. Many studies are under way to evaluate massage therapy further, including research on its effects in infants exposed to HIV, children with asthma, adolescents with eating disorders, adults with hypertension and patients recovering from surgery.

Massage can also aid people who cannot use their muscles actively because of injury, illness or paralysis. Although it cannot substitute for the normal muscular activity that rids the muscles of toxic products, massage can help the process when a person is unable to be normally active.

Preparations/Techniques

There are approximately 100 different methods of massage therapy, about 80 of them born in the period of revival since the mid-1970s. A simple classification includes traditional European methods, contemporary Western methods, energetic manual techniques and Oriental manual techniques.

The traditional European methods are based on longstanding Western concepts of anatomy and physiology. They use the five kinds of soft-tissue manipulation—effleurage, petrissage, friction, percussion, and vibration and jostling (the basic Swedish massage strokes)—illustrated in the Gallery of Massage Techniques that begins on page 95.

Contemporary Western methods add to the traditional techniques more recent knowledge of the effects of massage on the nervous system, posture, movement and emotion. Also included in contemporary methods are techniques such as Rolfing and the Alexander and Feldenkrais methods *(see Body Work, pages 35-44)* that are said to integrate the body in relationship to gravity.

Energetic and Oriental manual techniques use pressure and manipulation to assess, evaluate and balance the energy system said to surround and infuse the human body. Therapeutic touch *(page 43)* is an energetic technique. Oriental methods include shiatsu and acupressure *(pages 6-7)*.

Visiting a Professional

You can find a qualified massage therapist through a doctor's recommendation, a friend's advice (make sure the therapist belongs to a national organization),

CAUTION

Consult a doctor if you are considering massage therapy and have had an injury or a chronic illness such as heart or kidney disease. You should not use massage if you have an infection, inflammation or cancer that could spread throughout the body or if you have a blood clot. Massage is not appropriate for some cases of oedema because it can encourage more bleeding and swelling. If you have a nerve injury, you might find pressure on the skin painful. Do not use massage on your abdomen if you have high blood pressure or a peptic ulcer, and avoid massaging burned areas until they are healed.

CONTINUED

Massage CONTINUED

or by contacting the organization listed below, left. On your first visit, the massage therapist should ask about your medical history and current state of health in order to tailor the therapy to your particular problems.

You will probably need to disrobe completely or partially, depending on the areas to be worked on. The therapist will position you comfortably on a massage table and provide a sheet or large towel to drape over the areas of your body that are not being massaged. During your session, pay attention to your reactions and speak up if an area is painful or tender to the touch.

Doing It Yourself

If you are planning to practise massage with a partner, start with a few of the basic strokes and begin lightly, adding deeper strokes gradually. Wear loose clothing, remove your watch and rings, and keep your fingernails short to avoid scratching. Wash your hands thoroughly before beginning. Although shiatsu is done on the floor on a pad or futon, massage is best performed on a massage table. Keep the lighting gentle for optimum relaxation, and keep the room warm.

While massaging, keep your hands on your partner as much as possible, breaking contact gently and slowly to change areas. If your partner's muscles tighten, the pressure may be either too severe, causing discomfort, or too light, causing a tickling sensation. Do not massage directly a very tender area or the exact site of an injury. Put your body weight behind the pressure, rather than using your hands and arms alone, and keep your hands as relaxed as possible.

Well-being

The ability of massage to reduce stress and tension, tone muscles and enhance well-being makes it a useful part of a regular health maintenance programme. Athletes often use massage to prepare muscles for strenuous activity or to recover from it.

What the Critics Say

Some conventional practitioners worry that ill or injured people may seek massage in place of required medical treatment; however, massage therapists are usually knowledgeable about the need for conventional treatment. As with any therapy, patients should be wary of any extreme or quick-cure claims. ■

FOR MORE INFO

Following is an organization you can contact to learn more about massage therapy:

British Massage Therapy Council
Greenbank House
65a Adelphi Street
Preston PR1 7BG
01772 881 063

Shiatsu Society
Interchange Studios
Dalby Street
London NW5 3NQ
020 7813 7772

Effleurage

Massage of most areas of the body begins and ends with effleurage, a slow, rhythmic, gliding stroke performed with the fingertips, palms, thumbs, knuckles or whole hand. Generally, effleurage moves from the extremities towards the heart—from wrist to shoulder, for example. An exception is the nerve stroke, which does not affect blood flow and is done in the direction opposite to a preceding series of effleurage strokes.

Start lightly and gradually work deeper. You may end your massage of each area with the nerve stroke, which is particularly soothing. The broad surface of the back is ideal for practising the variations of effleurage pictured here. Keep your hands relaxed; tense, rigid hands have less sensitivity and don't feel as good to your partner.

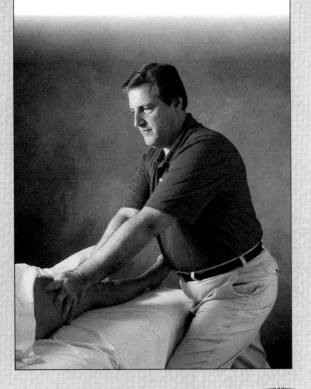

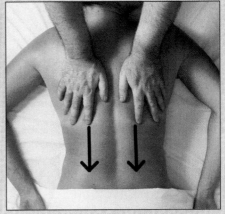

Basic Effleurage • Position your hands close together, with your thumbs 1–2 in (2.5–5 cm) apart. Stroke downward, keeping your hands in firm, full contact with your partner's body until you reach the top of the pelvic bone.

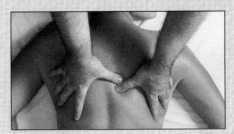

Adjacent Thumb • Place one thumb next to the other and glide down the back. Most of the pressure should be applied by your thumbs.

Posture • Align your body properly to prevent fatigue and strain. Use the entire weight of your upper body, rather than your hands alone, for pressure; the lower body should balance and support. In general, face the direction in which your hands are moving.

CONTINUED

Gallery of Massage Techniques

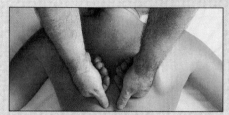

Loose Fist • Work large muscles with a loose fist, making contact with the area of the fingers between the second and third joints. Glide down the back.

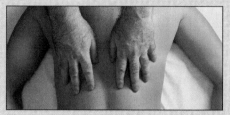

Nerve Stroke • While barely touching the skin, drag your fingertips up the back, moving in the reverse direction from previous effleurage strokes.

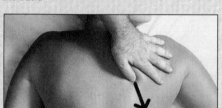

One Thumb • For a deeper stroke, use one thumb to glide deeply along smaller muscles. Use a little more pressure to contact muscles that lie underneath the superficial layers of muscle.

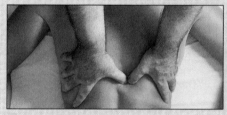

Joined Thumb • Place your thumbs along the erector muscles next to the spine. Starting just below the base of the neck, slide your thumbs down, using more pressure than with previous strokes.

Petrissage

A more complex technique, petrissage works specific muscle groups, usually where tissue is easily grasped. It can be performed deeply or superficially. Deep petrissage helps promote circulation and can counteract muscle tightness or degeneration. Alternately tighten and loosen your hands, fingers or thumbs as you pick up and release muscles. Variations include rolling, heel of palm and compression. Note the change in musculature as you go from tendons and ligaments towards the centre of a muscle, which can usually withstand more pressure.

Hand on Hand • Use this stroke on the abdomen. Place the fingers of your top hand over the bottom hand for support. Ask your partner to bend her knees. Proceed clockwise in a circle, exerting even pressure.

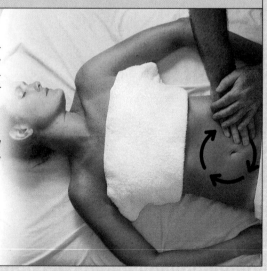

Gallery of Massage Techniques

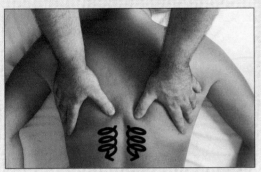

Spiral • *Pressing with both thumbs while making a sweeping motion, spiral down the back, using a counterclockwise motion with the left thumb and a clockwise motion with the right thumb. Go from the base of the neck to the waist.*

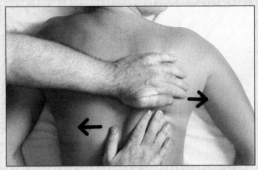

Rolling • *Slide your hand firmly back and forth across your partner's back. Push with the heel of one hand, and pull/lift the skin with the fingers of the other. Note how this stroke wrings the tissues between your two hands.*

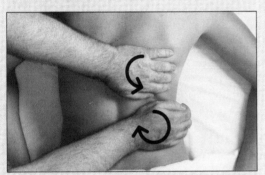

Heel of Palm • *Place the heels of your palms next to your partner's spine. Alternately rotating your palms in opposite directions, push the muscle gently away from the spine as you work down the back, so the muscle is kneaded but not pinched.*

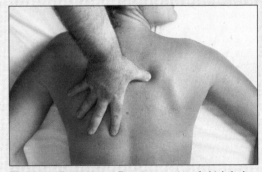

Direct Pressure • *For trigger points (which feel like small marbles), for knots of muscle tension, or to execute shiatsu techniques, press with the pad of your thumb or finger straight into the tissue. Hold for five to 15 seconds or until you feel the tension release.*

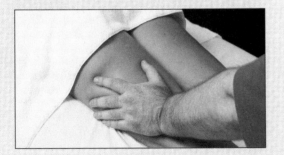

Compression • *Place one palm flat with the fingers relaxed. Pump your hand up and down rhythmically, directing the pressure toward the bone underneath, then releasing the pressure. Do not use this technique on joints.*

CONTINUED

Friction

Friction is often used in areas around joints. As in petrissage, you move muscle or other soft tissue away from bone. But in friction, the fingers or thumbs move over the underlying structures without sliding on the surface of the skin where the fingers or thumbs touch.

Because they have a relatively poor blood supply, tendons and ligaments tend to heal slowly, particularly during vigorous activities, sometimes resulting in 'overuse' syndromes. Friction increases circulation and helps restore range of motion; it is a mainstay of sports massage, where it is referred to as cross-fibre stroking. Use your fingertips and thumbs to perform friction; lighten pressure if your partner experiences discomfort. Friction should not be used on an area that has been injured within the past 24 to 48 hours.

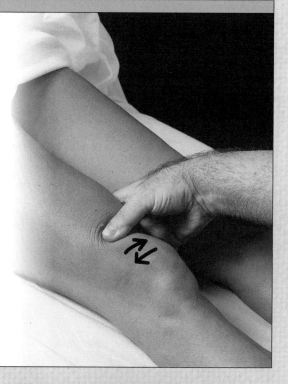

■ ***Cross-Fibre*** • *Pressing down, slide the thumb across the grain of the muscle (perpendicular to the muscle fibre) in a rhythmic motion. Keep your thumb on the same spot on the skin surface. You may feel the muscle fibres moving under your thumb.*

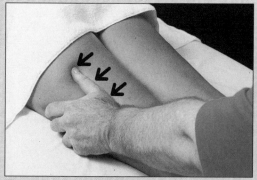

■ ***Broad Cross-Fibre Stroking*** • *Place your hand on the centre of the back of the leg. While applying pressure with the outside edge of your thumb and palm, stroke across the grain of the muscle of the entire outer leg. Switch hands, and repeat on the inner portion of the leg.*

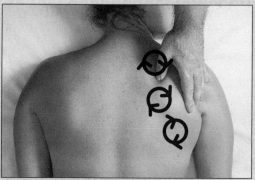

■ ***Circular Friction*** • *Locate the rope-like tissues that join the shoulder blade to the back. Using your hand for balance, place your thumb on the tissues and rotate it in small circles. Move down a bit, repeat the motion and continue until the entire area is covered.*

Percussion

Percussion strokes, also called tapotement (French for tapping), are alternate drumming hand movements performed on broad areas of the body, particularly the back. This stroke is clearly beneficial for increasing surface blood circulation, and it can help loosen phlegm and make it easier to expectorate it from the lungs.

When done properly, percussion is stimulating rather than painful or harsh. Keep your hands and wrists relaxed and elbows flexed. Strike the skin with alternating hands, moving rapidly over the surface you are working on. You should strike firmly but never so hard that you cause pain. Because even light percussion may cause discomfort to internal organs, do not apply it on the lower abdomen, the lower back near the kidneys, or directly on the spine.

Beating • Form a loose fist (inset) and strike gently with the outside surface. Beating works best on the fleshier areas of the body, such as the back, waist and thighs.

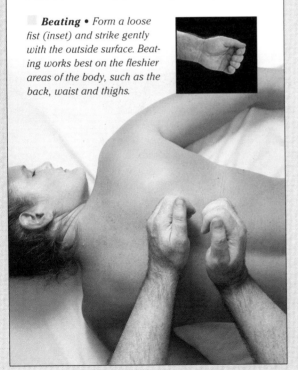

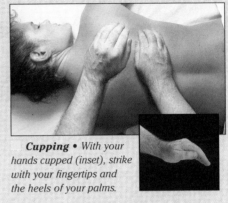

Cupping • With your hands cupped (inset), strike with your fingertips and the heels of your palms.

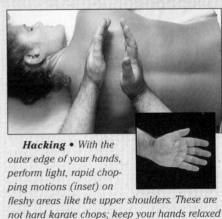

Hacking • With the outer edge of your hands, perform light, rapid chopping motions (inset) on fleshy areas like the upper shoulders. These are not hard karate chops; keep your hands relaxed with your fingers slightly separated.

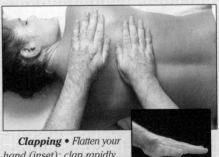

Clapping • Flatten your hand (inset); clap rapidly over fleshy areas like the upper back with the entire hand.

CONTINUED

Gallery of Massage Techniques

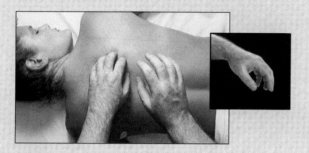

Tapping • Strike with the fingertips (inset), alternating your hands quickly. Unlike other percussion strokes, tapping may be helpful on bony areas such as the shoulder blades or scalp.

Vibration and Jostling

Like percussion, these techniques either stimulate or relax body tissue. The strokes are particularly effective on the limbs and fleshy areas. Vibration does not proceed in any specific direction; jostling works up and down a muscle.

Vibration requires a rapid contraction and relaxation of your own muscles, which sets up a vibratory wave that is transmitted to your partner through your hands. (Some professional massage therapists use mechanical vibrators for this effect.) One form of joint mobilization is a variation of vibration that uses larger motions to work the joints.

Jostling, which is not as strenuous, is used in sports massage, especially to treat sore muscles. If your partner's muscles tense up during massage, interrupt your sequence and relax the muscle area by jostling it for five or 10 seconds. You can insert jostling into a massage as often as you want.

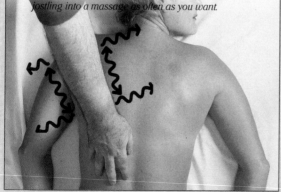

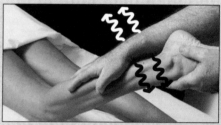

Jostling • Place your hands on your partner's calf and shake back and forth, progressing along the muscle.

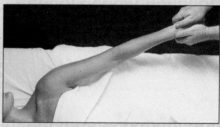

Joint Mobilization • Grasp your partner's hand firmly between your hands. Move far enough away so that your partner's arm is fully extended, and shake the arm with a wave-like motion while pulling away slightly from the joint.

Vibration • With your fingertips lightly touching your partner, tense all the muscles in your arm repeatedly, creating a trembling motion (left). The vibration you create in your arm is transferred through your fingers to the area being worked on.

Mind/Body Medicine

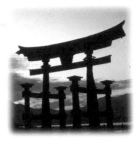

Close your eyes and imagine holding a freshly cut, bright yellow lemon in your hand. Imagine raising it to your mouth and biting into the tart pulp. The saliva now flooding your mouth is evidence of the powerful connection between the thoughts in your mind and the physical processes of your body.

Western science has long viewed the mind and the body as separate entities. Using increasingly sophisticated drugs and surgical techniques, doctors have focused on the body while almost wholly ignoring the mind's role in illness and healing. Yet the mind appears to have enormous influence on the progress of disease: Studies suggest that people's opinions about the state of their own health can dramatically affect their chances of developing a serious disease later in life.

Mind/body medicine seeks to explore connections between the tangible body and the intangible mind, and to use these linkages to improve physical as well as mental health. The techniques are not so much treatments as they are processes that help people learn how to influence their physical reactions. A common goal among the various mind/body techniques is relaxation, an important weapon in the modern battle against stress-related disease.

Target Ailments

- Back Problems
- Cancer
- Chronic Fatigue Syndrome
- Depression
- Diabetes
- Headache
- Heart Problems
- High Blood Pressure
- Immune Problems
- Incontinence
- Insomnia
- Irritable Bowel Syndrome
- Menopause Problems
- Menstrual Problems
- Pain, Chronic
- Seasonal Affective Disorder
- Stress
- TMJ Syndrome

Stress and Relaxation

The body reacts to stressful situations—sudden danger, for example—by releasing chemicals that produce a number of physical effects, such as an increase in heart rate, blood pressure and muscle tension. Chronic or long-term stress can take a serious toll. It suppresses immune system activity and can lead to insomnia, anxiety, high blood pressure, depression and possibly even cancer. Fortunately, the body has a recuperative reaction that can reverse many of the harmful effects of chronic stress: relaxation. Mind/body medicine is the quest to invoke the relaxation response and strengthen the body in pursuit of good health.

Mind/body techniques cannot replace conventional treatment, especially in the case of serious or chronic ailments, but they can be extremely useful as complementary therapies. Low in risk and cost, easy to learn, and adaptable to individual tastes, these methods can be combined and practised in a number of ways. They can be used in conjunction with conventional or other alternative therapies to control the symptoms of disease or the side effects of certain treatments, or they can be practised on a regular basis to promote and maintain overall health. And because they involve the active participation of the patient, mind/body techniques help foster a sense of control and self-reliance that in itself can be of significant therapeutic value.

CONTINUED

Mind/Body Medicine CONTINUED

The Power of the Patient

Medical science generally has not accepted mind/body medicine, perhaps because thoughts do not lend themselves readily to scientific testing methods. However, a number of mind/body therapies—meditation, guided imagery and prayer, for example—have been used successfully by traditional healers for hundreds of years. Even today, many doctors who do not embrace mind/body concepts acknowledge the influence the mind can have on disease. Some medical schools, in fact, teach the importance of a good bedside manner, realizing that what the patient believes about an illness—and also what the patient thinks the *doctor* believes—can change the course of the disease. The placebo effect is another familiar example of the curative power of belief. Convinced that a given medicine will bring relief, the patient actually does improve, even though the pills contain nothing but sugar.

The effectiveness of mind/body medicine depends largely on the level of patient commitment, as well as on the strength of one's belief that positive thinking can translate into better health. For these techniques to work, you must have realistic expectations and guidance from a competent, experienced therapist. Finding such a person may take some work, but the effort could pay off in long-term health benefits.

What the Critics Say

Despite evidence that the mind can and does play a role in healing, a number of healthcare professionals—even some who accept the general premise—remain sceptical of mind/body techniques. Some think that the benefits are limited, that patients will become frustrated if a technique does not produce significant improvements right away, or that patients will rely solely on mind/body techniques when other types of medical care are warranted. Many conventional doctors, for example, are concerned that patients using mind/body techniques will neglect to get proper, proven treatment for serious illnesses such as cancer, heart disease or diabetes. While mind/body methods are themselves safe and can often help people recover from disease, using them as substitutes for a doctor's care can delay necessary treatment and lead to serious problems.

Mind/body techniques also have come under attack because of possible dangers of receiving treatment from practitioners who are unlicensed or poorly qualified. For some of these therapies, practitioners are not required to pass an examination or get special training. This, say critics, opens the way for unscrupulous practitioners to take a patient's money and offer nothing in return but false hopes. And while proponents point to numerous studies showing that thoughts and deeply held beliefs can have a tremendous effect on one's health, some sceptics argue that the claims of mind/body medicine are not supported by scientific research.

Mind/Body Medicine

Biofeedback

In biofeedback, sensors on the body pick up electrical signals from the muscles or brain and pass them along to a computer, which translates the pulses into images or sounds. The patient watches or listens to these processed signals and, with the help of a therapist, develops ways to affect their rate or intensity. Eventually, the patient learns to exercise conscious control over normally unconscious bodily processes, such as blood pressure and heart rate.

What It's Good For • Biofeedback is used in many areas of medicine. It is especially helpful in the treatment of ailments that are caused or exacerbated by stress or anxiety, such as stress-induced hypertension and headaches. Many physical therapists use biofeedback to re-educate weak or overactive muscles, as well as to treat nerve damage and temporomandibular joint (TMJ) syndrome. Biofeedback may also be used to help reduce the frequency of epileptic seizures.

- **Headaches:** Biofeedback training is frequently recommended for the treatment of certain types of headaches.
- **Raynaud's syndrome:** Thermal, or temperature regulation, biofeedback is a successful therapy for this disorder, which causes cold feet and hands due to constricted blood vessels.
- **Attention deficit disorder:** One promising new form of biofeedback aims to teach people with this disorder how to normalize brain waves associated with concentration, attention and hyperactivity.
- **Diabetes:** Biofeedback training in relaxation techniques may help diabetics gain better metabolic control and learn to manage stress; stress can contribute to increased blood sugar levels in some people with the disease.

Visiting a Professional Biofeedback is best learned with the help of a healthcare professional who has experience using its techniques to treat your condition. Learning to access and then control the body's functions usually takes at least eight to 10 visits. Consult your doctor for a referral, or contact one of the organisations on the right for more information.

CAUTION

If you use a pacemaker or other implanted electrical aid or if you have a serious heart disorder, check with your physician before using a biofeedback device that measures the output of the sweat glands. These devices use a tiny amount of electricity, and although no problems have been reported with their use, several biofeedback organizations recommend this precaution.

FOR MORE INFO
Following is a list of organizations you can contact to learn more about biofeedback:

Biofeedback Foundation of Europe
PO Box 211
3440 AA Woerden
The Netherlands

Association for Applied Psychophysiology and Biofeedback
10200 West 44th Ave., Suite 304
Wheat Ridge, CO 80033-2840
USA

CONTINUED

Mind/Body Medicine

CAUTION

Guided imagery and hypnosis can be used as diagnostic tools in certain kinds of emotional therapy, sometimes involving the recovery of so-called repressed memories. In a number of cases, however, these memories, though seemingly quite real to both patient and therapist at the time of recovery, have been found to be false. This is an area where it pays to be careful and move slowly.

Guided Imagery

Guided imagery is a technique that uses the mind's ability to imagine sights, sounds, movements and other sensory experiences as a means to induce specific physical reactions in the body or to encourage changes in a patient's emotional outlook. Buddhists have used mental images to promote healing since the 13th century or earlier, and many shamanistic traditions around the world include the power of imagery. The technique can be used in many ways and can be adapted to suit different personalities; what doesn't work for one person might be the perfect therapy for another.

What It's Good For • Just as lying on a warm beach, listening to the ocean waves, and feeling the warm sunshine can have a relaxing effect on your body, so can visualizing such a scene in your mind. Similarly, imagining your immune cells as a conquering army or a swarm of victorious hunters may actually boost the cells' activity and, at the same time, promote a sense of self-reliance that further improves the functioning of your immune system. Simply relaxing and allowing images to take shape in your mind may give you insight into a symptom or ailment, and perhaps even suggest ideas about how to cope with it.

Guided imagery can have a profound influence on physical as well as psychological conditions. Studies of the brain indicate that merely imagining a certain activity stimulates the same regions of the cerebral cortex as actually experiencing the activity. This suggests that guided imagery has the potential to bring about positive physiological changes in the body, allowing a patient to exercise conscious control over such vital functions as heart rate, brain-wave rhythms and blood glucose levels.

A number of natural childbirth groups rely on a type of preparatory guided imagery called mental rehearsal, in which women imagine going through delivery before the actual event. Mental rehearsal is also frequently used by patients as a way to relieve anxiety before surgery. This sort of preview can reduce pain and side effects, and even shorten recovery time.

■ **Immune problems:** A number of studies show improvement in some immune reactions following imagery training. Sometimes guided imagery is combined with other mind/body techniques to boost the effectiveness of the immune system.

■ **Cancer:** Guided imagery is often used by cancer patients in an effort to mobilize their immune system against the disease. There is no direct evidence that imagery alone can improve the prognosis, but people often report that imagery

Mind/Body Medicine

makes them better able to cope with cancer. Studies have shown that imagery can also ease nausea and promote weight gain in cancer patients undergoing treatments that interfere with their eating habits.

- **Irritable bowel syndrome:** Using guided imagery to visualize a soothing scene or activity can help relieve the symptoms of IBS.
- **Asthma:** Guided imagery may help asthma patients relax and assume better control of their breathing.

Preparations/Techniques • Guided imagery can be used actively—as when a cancer patient imagines immune cells attacking malignant cells—or receptively, allowing the mind to form images that might shed light on a particular ailment or condition. Techniques for both approaches can be learned on your own from a book or an audiotape, or under the guidance of a trained therapist.

Taking the time to concentrate on observing the world around you helps your mind create more convincing images. Clarity is important for healing, because the more vivid the image, the more 'real' it seems and the greater its effect on the nervous system. While conjuring 'pictures' is perhaps the easiest form of imagery, it is also possible—and equally relaxing—to imagine soothing sounds, sensations of touch and smells. For chronic conditions, guided imagery is most beneficial when practised for 15 or 20 minutes once or twice every day. You may want to keep a journal of your sessions and your symptoms to help you evaluate the results. Guided imagery for relaxation can be used regularly or on the spur of the moment—to handle a tense situation or cope with sudden pain, for example.

Visiting a Professional • Many kinds of therapists use guided imagery, and some teach individuals or groups how to continue its use on their own. It may take several sessions with a professional and some time working on your own before you notice results. Ask your doctor for a referral to a therapies.

Well-being • Guided imagery can help you picture well-being or success in any number of endeavours. Using imagery to take mini-holidays throughout the day can keep you relaxed and help prevent or tone down the stress response.

FOR MORE INFO
Following is a list of organizations you can contact to learn more about guided imagery:

The Academy for Guided Imagery
PO Box 2070
Mill Valley, CA 94942
USA
fax: (415) 389-9342

The Institute of Transpersonal Psychology
744 San Antonio Road
Palo Alto, CA 94303
USA
fax: (650) 493-6835

CONTINUED

Mind/Body Medicine CONTINUED

Hypnotherapy

Healers have used hypnotism to induce trance states in patients since ancient times. Although the practice has largely fallen out of favour among mainstream doctors, over the last few decades a number of healthcare practitioners in various fields have begun to harness the power of hypnotherapy to treat an array of conditions.

What It's Good For • Hypnotherapy aims to induce a state of focused concentration, described as neither sleep nor wakefulness, during which a willing subject is open and responsive to suggestion. (An unwilling subject cannot be hypnotized.) Hypnotherapy is most effective when used to treat ailments involving stress or anxiety. There are also reports of success with hypnotherapy in helping people break bad habits, such as bedwetting in children, or establish good ones.

- **Skin problems:** Hypnotherapy has been used successfully to treat warts and ichthyosis (fish skin disease), a severe genetic disorder.
- **Pain:** Some doctors, dentists and midwives use hypnotherapy to counteract the fear and anxiety that can heighten pain, complicate healing, and slow labour in women giving birth. Clinical trials also show that hypnotherapy can help burn patients deal more effectively with pain.
- **Haemophilia:** Research shows that hypnotherapy may reduce bleeding in people with this disorder, which interferes with the blood's ability to form clots.
- **Anxiety:** Hypnotherapy can help people overcome certain phobias, including stage fright, or cope with distressing situations such as hospitalization.

Visiting a Professional • A trained therapist can guide you through the steps of hypnosis or teach you how to perform the techniques yourself. Ask your doctor for a referral to a qualified therapist, or contact a national organization *(left)*.

Wellness • Hypnosis is thought to bring about physiological changes similar to those induced by other relaxation techniques. It also offers the same potential for increased overall well-being and helps to prevent or reduce the intensity of the stress response.

CAUTION

Hypnotic suggestions can be very powerful. Before undergoing hypnotherapy, make sure that your practitioner is qualified and has experience in treating your particular condition.

FOR MORE INFO

Following areorganizations you can contact to learn more about hypnotherapy:

British Hypnotherapy Association
67 Upper Berkeley Street
London W1H 7DH
020 7723 4443

National Register of Hypnotherapists & Psychotherapists
12 Cross Street
Nelson
Lancashire BB9 7EN
01282 699 378
fax: 01282 698 633
email: Hypnosis_NCHP@ compuserve.com

Mind/Body Medicine

Meditation

Many cultures throughout the world have recognized the calming, therapeutic effect of quiet contemplation. Most types of meditation practised today, however, come from ancient Eastern or other religious traditions. Almost all of these methods share a few simple steps. Students are instructed to sit quietly, usually with eyes closed, and focus the mind on a single thought, allowing all other thoughts to float away. Some forms are more active or complex, meant to be performed while walking or chanting, for example.

One of the most famous methods is transcendental meditation, or TM, a simplified variation of ancient yoga that was brought to the West by Maharishi Mahesh Yogi in the 1960s. Another type is known as the relaxation response (pages 109-110). A traditional Buddhist method called vipassana, or mindfulness meditation, has been practised in the East for 2,500 years but only recently become known to the Western world. Students of mindfulness meditation are taught simply to focus on the present moment. The goal is to face and accept all aspects of life, thereby achieving a deeper sense of balance that contributes to overall well-being.

What It's Good For • Meditation is commonly thought of as a spiritual endeavour, but it has frequently demonstrated physical effects as well. Most forms of meditation promote regular quiet relaxation, which in itself can help alleviate symptoms of stress-related ailments ranging from headaches to high blood pressure.

- **Chronic pain:** Use of TM or mindfulness meditation has been shown to reduce the suffering associated with chronic pain, possibly by helping people examine and sort out the negative thoughts commonly generated during intense discomfort.
- **High blood pressure:** Studies have shown a decrease in blood pressure among regular practitioners of TM. This evidence is so persuasive that cardiologists sometimes recommend meditation to their patients to help lower stress-related hypertension.
- **Stress:** TM has been used in treating post-traumatic stress disorder. Recent studies suggest a connection between meditation and a decrease in the levels of harmful stress-induced chemicals in the brain. Mindfulness meditation has been shown to reduce anxiety, depression and other symptoms associated with stress.
- **Panic disorders:** Mindfulness meditation can help people prone to panic attacks control their breathing and reactions, thereby forestalling full attacks.

CAUTION

Some people experience disorientation and anxiety when beginning to meditate. To overcome feelings like these, try keeping your eyes open and focusing your attention on a picture or an object. You can also learn to meditate while walking. Discuss such problems with your instructor, therapist or doctor.

CONTINUED

Mind/Body Medicine CONTINUED

- **Headaches:** The relaxation achieved through meditation can help reduce or eliminate headaches brought on by stress or muscle tension.
- **Respiratory problems:** For some patients with emphysema, asthma or other lung ailments, mindfulness meditation can reduce the frequency and severity of attacks of breathlessness.

Preparations/Techniques • Meditation seems simple, but learning to stop the usual stream of conscious thoughts flowing through your mind takes practice. First, you must find a quiet place with as few distractions as possible. Sit quietly in a comfortable position, preferably with your back straight. Focus your mind on your breath or on a silently repeated sound, word or phrase (called a mantra), or on a stationary object such as a flower or candle flame. If other thoughts intrude, take notice of them, but then let them go and return your focus to the phrase or object. Gently refocus as many times as necessary. Practise this for 15 to 20 minutes twice a day; meditating at the same time every day helps reinforce the habit.

For mindfulness meditation, begin the same way, using a single point of concentration to achieve calm. When thoughts or feelings surface, observe them without intention or judgment; don't try to decide if your thoughts are right or wrong, just be aware of them. The goal of this form of meditation is acceptance of the reality of the moment. For a technique known as the body scan, performed while seated or lying down, concentrate on moving your attention through your body, taking note of any sensations or impressions as you go along.

Although it is possible to learn to meditate on your own with the help of instruction books or courses on audiotape or videotape, it is best to begin with a qualified instructor. Classes and retreats in the various methods are widely available; many people, in fact, find that the support of others in a group setting provides the motivation necessary for developing the proper meditation skills.

Well-being • Many who practise meditation say that the relaxation and focus provided by regular sessions positively affects every aspect of life. Mindfulness meditation, in particular, appears to foster a sense of connection that promotes general good health and may actually bring about beneficial changes in specific areas of the body, including the cardiovascular system.

FOR MORE INFO

Following is an organization you can contact to learn more about meditation:

The Kevala Centre
Hunsdon Road
Torquay
Devon TQ1 1QB
01803 215 678
email: information@kevala.co.uk
website: www. kevala.co.uk

Mind/Body Medicine

Relaxation Techniques

In the late 1960s, Harvard cardiologist Herbert Benson became intrigued by the incidence of high blood pressure in patients who were under stress. While researching this phenomenon, he noticed that blood pressure levels were lower in people who meditated than in those who didn't. Eventually, he identified a mechanism in the body that helps reduce stress. This mechanism, which Benson called the relaxation response, can be invoked in a number of ways. Yoga (pages 141-142), t'ai chi (pages 139-140), and qigong (pages 134-135), for example, are excellent techniques for promoting relaxation and reducing stress. Others include the relaxation methods listed on page 110 in 'Preparations/Techniques'. These simple techniques can be used virtually anywhere at any time, and most of them need no special training, just practice.

CAUTION

Relaxation methods can reduce your need for certain medications. Whatever technique you decide to use, keep your doctor informed so he or she can make any necessary adjustments in dosage.

What It's Good For • Relaxation is the goal of mind/body medicine because it helps reduce the negative effects of stress, which has been linked to many serious and chronic diseases, including cancer, heart disease and depression. Summoning the relaxation response also lowers the respiration rate and relaxes muscle tension. One researcher found that regular use of relaxation techniques makes the body less responsive throughout the day to the effects of noradrenaline, a stress hormone that increases blood pressure and heart rate. Relaxation training may also be helpful after surgery or other medical procedures. Research suggests that using these techniques may speed healing, reduce bleeding and other complications, decrease pain and reliance on medications and perhaps allow a quicker return to full health.

- **Insomnia:** Learning to evoke the relaxation response can help many people with chronic insomnia improve their ability to fall asleep. A technique referred to as progressive muscle relaxation (*page 110*) is a particularly beneficial way to promote deep, all-body relaxation and to overcome sleeplessness.
- **Premenstrual syndrome:** Symptoms of PMS were significantly reduced in women who practised relaxation techniques twice a day for three months.
- **Immune problems:** Studies show an increase in immune cell activity after relaxation training.
- **High blood pressure:** Relaxation techniques are very effective in lowering elevated blood pressure in cases of stress-related hypertension.
- **Infertility:** Stress can interfere with the normal hormonal cycle of the reproductive process in women, sometimes resulting in infertility. In one study, a group of women thought to be infertile participated in relaxation training, and

CONTINUED

Mind/Body Medicine CONTINUED

a third of them became pregnant. Relaxation techniques can also help alleviate the stress associated with the experience of infertility or its treatment.

Preparations/Techniques • Herbert Benson suggests the following technique for triggering the relaxation response. Sit comfortably in a place with minimal distractions. Close your eyes and relax your muscles. Breathe naturally; as you exhale, silently repeat a word or phrase you have chosen that has meaning to you—this is your 'focus word'. Many people use 'peace' or 'love', a short prayer, or the name of a religious figure as a focus word. Remain passive; when other thoughts intrude, let them go and return to your focus word. Continue to concentrate for 10 to 20 minutes, then open your eyes and sit quietly for a moment before you get up. Practise this technique once or twice a day.

Another method, which is called progressive muscle relaxation, involves concentrating on each muscle group in the body, one at a time, and moving progressively from one end of the body to the other. Inhale and clench your muscles for five seconds, then exhale and relax. Repeat for each area of your body until your entire body is relaxed.

A technique called autogenic training combines relaxation with self-hypnosis and guided imagery. Autogenic training involves the repetition of meaningful phrases to yourself while focusing on a sense of heaviness and warmth in the limbs, breathing calmly and keeping the muscles limp and relaxed.

A number of relaxation techniques, including yoga and moving meditation, focus on the breath. Deep breathing can release tension and speed delivery of oxygen to the body and relax the nervous system. Breathing exercises can be done anywhere at any time and are easily combined with most other relaxation methods.

Well-being • Habitual use of relaxation techniques rests and recharges the body, thereby strengthening it against daily or unusual stress. Quietening the mind may also promote greater concentration and receptivity to information, suggesting that relaxation techniques can foster good health and boost overall well-being.

FOR MORE INFO
Contact the following organization to learn more about relaxation techniques:

The Kevala Centre
Hunsdon Road
Torquay
Devon TQ1 1QB
01803 215 678
email: information@kevala.co.uk
website: www.kevala.co.uk

Mind/Body Medicine

Spiritual Healing and Prayer

Almost every culture, society and religious tradition throughout history has acknowledged the healing power of faith and prayer.

What It's Good For • Religious belief and prayer bring comfort, hope and relaxation to the faithful of all backgrounds. Studies have shown that regular spiritual observance, prayer and religious ritual are beneficial to overall health.

- **Heart problems:** In one study showing the power of intercessory prayer, a group of heart patients for whom strangers had secretly prayed were found to have fewer complications than another group of patients who did not receive the prayers of others.
- **Addiction:** Many treatment programmes use the concept of a 'higher power' to help people refrain from substance abuse or other bad habits.
- **Terminal illness:** Spirituality and religion help dying patients cope with the prospect of death, especially as they search for meaning in their lives and in their suffering.

Preparations/Techniques • People of various faiths pray in different ways, and the style of prayer can differ vastly even among people who attend the same place of worship. Believers do not need a deity to pray, nor does prayer require words; certain feelings, such as compassion, and even silent contemplation of the infinite are also considered types of prayer. For some, it may be best to surrender health problems to a higher power and trust in the outcome, rather than to pray for a specific result.

Well-being • Spiritual belief can help people transcend sickness or pain and achieve a sense of health and well-being. To experience the healing effects of spirituality does not require religious adherence, though religious commitment can have positive effects. Rather, it demands nothing more than an ability to love, to forgive, and to seek meaning and purpose beyond the circumstances of the moment. ∎

CAUTION

Beware of any healer who promises a complete cure of a serious illness without the use of conventional diagnostic or therapeutic methods. Faith and prayer can be powerful medicine, but for many diseases their role should be considered supportive or complementary.

FOR MORE INFO

Following areorganizations you can contact to learn more about spiritual healing:

National Federation of Spiritual Healers
Old Manor Farm Studio
Church Street
Sunbury on Thames
Middlesex TW16 6RG

Great World Spiritual Healing Fellowship
Greater World Spiritual Centre
3–5 Conway Street
London W1P 5HA
020 7436 7555

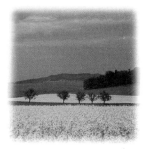

$\mathcal{N}$aturopathic Medicine

Target Ailments

- Allergies
- Arthritis
- Asthma
- Back Problems
- Cholesterol Problems
- Constipation
- Depression
- Headache
- Heartburn
- High Blood Pressure
- Insomnia
- Menstrual Problems
- Nausea
- Pain, Chronic
- Stress

N *aturopathic medicine aims to provide holistic, or whole-body, healthcare by drawing from numerous traditional healing systems. At its core is the idea of vis medicatrix naturae—the healing power of nature. Naturopathic doctors believe that the body naturally strives for health and that the doctor's role is to support the body's efforts. To achieve this, naturopaths follow seven basic principles: Help nature heal, do no harm, find the underlying cause, treat the whole person, encourage prevention, recognize well-being and act as a teacher.*

A naturopathic doctor, or ND, may pay considerable attention to a patient's lifestyle, since naturopathic theory holds that physical, psychological and even spiritual elements can all contribute to disease. In treating patients the naturopathic practitioner might use a number of alternative therapies, including homoeopathy, herbal remedies, Chinese medicine, spinal manipulation, nutrition, hydrotherapy, massage and exercise.

Origins

Although its origins trace to ancient times, naturopathy as a modern system of healing began in 1902, when German immigrant Benedict Lust founded the American School of Naturopathy in New York City. Having been cured of a debilitating condition by hydrotherapy, Lust became convinced that 'nature cures' were the best approach to well-being. His school grew rapidly, and by 1919 the American Naturopathic Association, also founded by Lust, was incorporated in 19 states. The movement flourished in the twenties and thirties, with thousands of practitioners attending national conventions and naturopathic journals and books gaining a growing audience. By the 1990s many of naturopathy's practices regarding diet, exercise, and lifestyle had become accepted by the wider medical community.

What It's Good For

Because of its emphasis on whole-body health, and with its wide range of techniques, naturopathy may be used for almost all basic healthcare. Patients visit naturopathic doctors for preventive care or for alternative therapies when conventional approaches have been unsatisfactory. Naturopaths have reported success with conditions such as chronic infections, fatigue and menstrual and menopausal problems. Diseases that are strongly affected by lifestyle and environment are among those most commonly treated by naturopaths. In a typical case of high blood pressure, for example, an ND might suggest a multifaceted approach involving changed diet, vitamin and mineral supplements, herbal medicines and lifestyle modifica-

Naturopathic Medicine

tions. For an arthritis sufferer, the primary treatments could include diet, homoeopathic medicines, acupuncture, hydrotherapy and massage. Naturopathic doctors also provide counselling for emotional and mental problems, such as depression and anxiety.

Visiting a Professional

Naturopathic doctors are usually surgery-based primary-care providers. Their approaches and treatments depend on their background and philosophy. Some stick to a strict 'natural' regimen of diet, detoxification and hydrotherapy; others may differ from conventional doctors only in using herbal medicines instead of synthetic drugs. Some naturopathic doctors specialize in a particular form of alternative medicine such as homoeopathy or acupuncture; others are generalists.

A first visit might take an hour, during which the doctor conducts a standard physical exam, possibly including conventional laboratory tests and radiology. In addition, the doctor will spend considerable time taking a patient history, assessing every aspect of the person's lifestyle, including diet, exercise, stress, and mental, emotional and spiritual issues.

After the initial evaluation, doctor and patient work together to establish a treatment programme. Because naturopathy emphasizes non-invasive therapies, the doctor will probably suggest ways the patient can change disease-promoting habits, help set realistic goals and identify the causes of unhealthy behaviour.

If the patient has a specific complaint, the doctor may prescribe any one of many natural treatments or a combination of those treatments. These could include nutrition, homoeopathic remedies, massage, botanical medicines, physical medicine (body work), hydrotherapy, acupuncture or psychological and family counselling. The naturopath may also prescribe conventional drugs, give vaccinations or perform outpatient surgery. In general, though, the aim of naturopathy is not only to cure a particular ailment but also to aid the body in sustaining lifelong good health.

Well-being

Well-being is what naturopathic medicine is all about. Naturopathic doctors believe that the body has an innate intelligence that strives for health; the role of both patient and doctor is to work with the body to help it promote its own well-being. Health, therefore, is more than the absence of disease; it is a vital state that needs encouragement and the proper environment. These doctors point out, for instance, that the substantial decline in deaths from heart attacks in recent decades is due not to improved coronary surgery but to public education regarding nutrition, exercise, and stress. In naturopathy, doctor and patient together will not only correct

113

CONTINUED

Naturopathic Medicine

imbalances and states of disease but also plan a lifelong course of diet, exercise and mental attitude that is designed to support the body's natural processes and fend off chronic disease and the debilitation normally associated with ageing.

What the Critics Say

Many members of the conventional medical establishment criticize naturopathy as being overly vague, too dependent on nutritional counselling and untested herbal remedies, and not subject to the scientific methods of experimentation and peer review. They say that the placebo effect is responsible for many of naturopathy's positive results. Critics also point out that almost anyone can get a mail-order naturopathy degree. Accredited NDs also acknowledge this danger and are attempting to persuade governments to establish standards for naturopathic doctors throughout the world. ■

FOR MORE INFO

Following is a list of organizations you can contact to learn more about naturopathy:

General Council & Register of Naturopaths
Frazer House
6 Netherhall Gardens
London NW3 5RR
website: www.naturopathy.org.uk

General Council and Register of Naturopaths
Goswell House
2 Goswell Road
Street
Somerset BA16 0JG
01458 840 072
fax: 01458 840 075

General Osteopathic Council Statutory Register
Premier House
10 Greycoat Place
London SW1P 1SB
website: www.osteopathy.org.uk

Nutrition and Diet

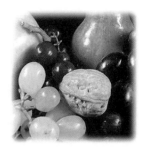

Eating a balanced diet is a major factor in a healthy lifestyle. Your body requires more than 40 nutrients for energy, growth and tissue maintenance. Water, as the most plentiful component in the body, is also crucial to survival. It is the medium for bodily fluids, and it transports nutrients into cells and carries waste products and toxins out.

Conventional and alternative practitioners alike acknowledge the importance of a healthy diet. Alternative practitioners, however, place more emphasis on dietary intervention in some conditions where conventional medicine would turn first to drugs or even surgery. Treatment of atherosclerosis, for example, may take the form of an extremely low-fat diet with a programme of meditation, exercise and support-group therapy.

Basic Nutrition

Carbohydrates, proteins and fats—macronutrients or 'energy nutrients'—provide fuel in the form of calories. Carbohydrates, the body's main energy source, are divided into two types. Simple carbohydrates are sugars, such as cane sugar and treacle; complex carbohydrates include starches, such as those found in potatoes and whole grains.

Proteins support tissue growth and repair, and help to produce antibodies, hormones and enzymes, which are essential for all the body's chemical reactions. Protein sources include meat, fish, dairy products, poultry, dried beans, nuts and eggs.

Dietary fat protects internal organs, provides energy, insulates against cold, and helps the body absorb certain vitamins. There are three kinds of fats: saturated, found in meat, dairy products, and coconut oil; monounsaturated, in olive and peanut oils; and polyunsaturated, in corn, cottonseed, safflower, sesame, soya bean and sunflower oils.

Your diet also supplies the important micronutrients we call vitamins and minerals. They are needed only in trace amounts, but the absence or deficiency of just one can cause major illness. With a few exceptions, the body does not manufacture micronutrients and so must obtain them from food.

Vitamins and minerals are essential for health. The European Community has determined a recommended daily allowance (RDA) for nineteen of the most important vitamins and minerals, but there are others which many nutritionists consider vital for a complete and healthy diet. *(See pages 123-133 for detailed information and recommended daily allowances, where applicable, for specific vitamins and minerals.)*

CONTINUED

Nutrition and Diet

Your body also needs dietary fibre, the indigestible part of plant foods. A high-fibre diet reduces the risks of various gastrointestinal problems, promotes cardiovascular health and may help decrease the risk of breast cancer and bowel cancer.

Diet Planning

In general, we eat more fat, protein, cholesterol, sugar and salt than we need. The following are some basic recommendations, based on official diet guidelines established by agencies in Britain and the United States:

OF SPECIAL INTEREST

Butter, Margarine or Olestra?

There is little question that limiting your intake of fat to 30 per cent of your daily calories or less is good for your health. But what kind of fats should you use? For decades, margarine has been recommended to replace butter and lard, which contain saturated fats. But margarine contains what are called trans fatty acids, which can contribute to a higher risk of heart disease. Olestra (chemically known as sucrose polyester, or SPE) is a fat substitute that provides no calories at all, and may appear to be the answer to a dieter's prayers. However,. although approved for use in the US, it has not been granted a license in the UK. Researchers have found that olestra could interfere with the absorption of some nutrients (including vitamin E and carotenoids) and drugs, and it may cause severe abdominal cramping, diarrhoea and vomiting in certain individuals.

Remember that some fat is essential to a well-balanced diet. Choose monounsaturated oils over saturated fats whenever possible.

- **Eat a variety of foods:** This will help ensure that you get the calories, protein, fibre, vitamins, minerals and other nutrients you need.
- **Control your weight:** Keep within recommended weight limits for your age, sex and build.
- **Eat a low-fat, low-cholesterol diet:** Ideally, no more than 30 per cent of your daily calories should come from fat, and no more than 10 per cent should come from saturated fat.
- **Eat plenty of vegetables, fruits and grains:** More than half of your daily calories should come from carbohydrates, rich in nutrients and low in fats; 80 per cent of those calories should be from complex carbohydrates.
- **Eat sugar and salt in moderation:** Sugar is high in calories and promotes tooth decay. Too much salt may increase the risk of developing high blood pressure. Prepared foods are notoriously high in salt or other forms of sodium, so check labels.
- **If you drink alcohol, do so in moderation:** Alcohol

Nutrition and Diet

provides calories but no nutrients, and too much is harmful. However, some studies indicate that moderate consumption of red wine may actually lower the risk of heart disease. 'Moderation' generally means one drink a day for women or two drinks for men.

Nutritional Supplements

If you consistently eat a well-balanced diet of fresh fruits, vegetables, grains and some animal protein, you probably don't require a nutritional supplement. Multinutrient supplements offer insurance for those times when eating well is a challenge—and can be indispensable during pregnancy or when you are ill, injured or under great mental or physical strain.

Generally, vitamins and minerals are recommended for daily use as a preventive measure. Supplements do, however, figure in the dietary recommendations of many therapies. Orthomolecular medicine, a form of nutrient therapy, uses combinations of vitamins, minerals and amino acids normally found in the body to treat specific conditions such as asthma, heart disease, depression, and schizophrenia. Such therapy can also be used to maintain general good health.

Taking vitamins or minerals in excess can upset the natural balance of nutrients. The fat-soluble vitamins—A, D, E and K—can be retained in your body and may be toxic in high amounts. The rest are water soluble and are unlikely to be toxic; excess amounts are excreted in the urine. Always take supplements in moderation; they are safe in doses at or below RDAs, but higher doses may be harmful and should be taken only under the guidance of a doctor or dietitian.

Supplement doses are measured by weight in milligrams (mg), or thousandths of a gram; in micrograms (mcg), or millionths of a gram; or in a universal standard known as international units (IU).

Food Allergies and Sensitivities

Some people cannot tolerate certain foods or food additives; the most common culprits include dairy products, soya beans, peanuts, wheat, eggs and shellfish. Allergic reactions can be very severe, even causing death, whereas sensitivities can cause troublesome symptoms such as rashes or bloating. Food intolerance may even be a factor in hyperactivity and many chronic diseases such as rheumatoid arthritis.

An elimination diet can help you pin down what food or foods are causing the reaction, and banning the offenders from your diet is one way to deal with this problem. A controversial method called desensitizing aims to train the body to accept foods it would otherwise not tolerate. One fairly common intolerance, that for milk sugar, can be addressed by adding a specific enzyme to the diet or by limiting the intake of dairy products to those, such as yoghurt, that are more easily digested.

FOR MORE INFO

Following is a list of organizations you can contact to learn more about nutrition and diet:

Food Commission
94 White Lion Street
London N1 9PF
020 7837 2250
fax: 020 7837 1141

Organic Living Association
St Mary's Villa
Hanley
Swan
Worcester WR8 0EA

Vegetarian Society
Parkdale
Dunham Road
Altrincham
Cheshire WA14 4QG
0161 928 0793
fax: 0161 926 9182
email: info@vegxoc.demon.co.uk

CONTINUED

Nutrition and Diet continued

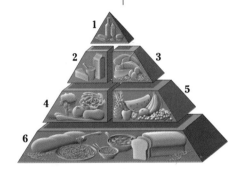

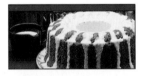

1 Fats, Oils & Sweets Group
USE SPARINGLY

One teaspoon (5 ml) of butter, oil, or margarine is a single serving.

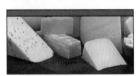

2 Milk, Yoghurt & Cheese Group
2-3 SERVINGS

One serving equals 8 fl oz (235 ml) milk/yoghurt, 1½ oz (45 g)natural cheese, 2 oz (60 g) processed cheese.

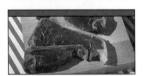

3 Meat, Poultry, Fish, Dried Beans, Eggs & Nuts Group   2-3 SERVINGS

One serving is 2–3 oz (60–85 g) of cooked lean meat, poultry, or fish. 1 oz (30 g) of meat equals one egg or 4 fl oz (120 ml) cooked dried beans.

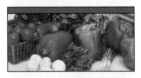

4 Vegetable Group
3-5 SERVINGS

One serving equals 8 fl oz (235 ml) of raw leafy greens, 4 fl oz (120 ml) of other vegetables or 6 fl oz (175 ml)of vegetable juice.

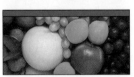

5 Fruit Group
2-4 SERVINGS

One serving is equal to one apple, orange or banana; 4 fl oz (120 ml) of chopped, cooked or canned fruit or 6 fl oz (175 ml) of fruit juice.

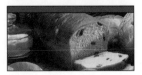

6 Bread, Cereal, Rice & Pasta Group
6-11 SERVINGS

One serving equals one slice of bread; half a bun, bagel or muffin; 1 oz (30 g) of dry cereal; or 4 fl oz (120 ml) of cooked cereal, rice or pasta.

T he Food Guide Pyramid—developed on the advice of nutritional scientists—makes healthy eating easier by showing how much of each type of food you should eat for good nutrition. Each of the groups provides some of the nutrients you need each day; no one group provides them all. Variety within and among groups is key.

The foundation of the pyramid is grain-based foods, which provide complex carbohydrates, vitamins, minerals and fibre. On the next level are fruits and vegetables, which are rich in vitamins, minerals and fibre but low in fat. The next two groups are critical sources of protein, calcium, iron, zinc and other nutrients, but many of these foods are also high in fat and cholesterol. Fats, oils and sweets occupy the tip of the pyramid and should be eaten sparingly.

The pyramid suggests a range of daily servings for each group. Your actual needs depend on your daily caloric requirements. Experts recommend about 1,600 calories for older adults and sedentary women; 2,200 calories for children, teenage girls, active women and sedentary men; and 2,800 calories for teenage boys, active men and very active women.

Nutrition and Diet

Below and on the following pages are descriptions of four diets, two of which (Asian and Mediterranean) are based on the traditional eating habits of certain cultures. All four plans are reported to have specific health benefits and may be recommended to help treat or prevent specific ailments.

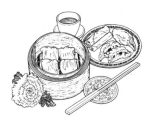

Asian Diet

People in Japan, Korea, South-east Asia and China have traditionally eaten a diet largely composed of rice, soya bean products and fresh vegetables, with little meat or dairy products. This diet is low in fat and high in complex carbohydrates.

What It's Good For

Besides generally avoiding saturated fats, the traditional Asian diet promotes good health in other ways.

- **Cancer:** Rice is high in protease inhibitors, substances believed to retard cancer. High consumption of rice is linked to low rates of some cancers, including bowel, breast and prostate. Soya beans also contain protease inhibitors; a study showed that consumption of one bowl a day of miso (soya bean paste) soup lowered risk of stomach cancer by almost a third.

  Sea vegetables are also included in the Japanese diet, and they appear to have anti-cancer properties as well. Oriental green tea exhibits anti-mutagenic properties and lowers rates of stomach cancer in people who drink it regularly.

- **Atherosclerosis:** Regular consumption of soy foods confers many health benefits, including lower blood cholesterol levels and less risk of atherosclerosis.

Preparations/Techniques

A diet based on Asian practices would include lots of rice—especially steamed—and soya bean foods, commonly tofu and miso; fresh vegetables and seaweed, steamed or stir-fried; fresh fruit; moderate amounts of fish; and very little red meat or other animal products, including dairy products. Important seasonings are garlic, ginger and soy sauce.

What the Critics Say

As with all diets that minimize animal proteins, a wide variety of foods and attention to menu planning are essential.

CONTINUED

Nutrition and Diet CONTINUED

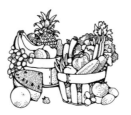

Macrobiotic Diet

From the Greek words for 'long' and 'life', the macrobiotic diet is based on a system taught by Japanese educator and philosopher George Ohsawa in the early 20th century. The diet eliminates all animal products except a small amount of fish, and emphasizes whole grains and cooked vegetables. Foods are described as *yin* (contractive) or *yang* (expansive), with a balance sought between the two. Foods that are excessively one or the other are excluded.

What It's Good For

Studies suggest that this diet's emphasis on whole grains and vegetables, and its elimination of processed foods, may have healthy effects on the body.

- **Heart disease:** Low in fat and high in complex carbohydrates and fibre, the macrobiotic diet promotes cardiovascular health.
- **Cancer:** There is evidence that a macrobiotic diet may lower the risk of breast cancer, and indeed the diet includes foods, such as soya bean products and sea vegetables, that contain cancer-fighting compounds. Use of a macrobiotic diet to help treat cancer is, however, controversial *(see What the Critics Say, below)*.

Preparations/Techniques

A macrobiotic diet prescribes deriving about 50 per cent of the diet from whole cereal grains; 20 to 30 per cent from vegetables; 5 to 10 per cent from beans and sea vegetables; and 5 to 10 per cent from soups. Occasional foods include fish—white-meat fish such as flounder and sole are recommended—fruits and nuts.

Foods to be avoided include potatoes, peppers, meat products, eggs, warm drinks, hot spices and any refined, mass-produced or artificially treated food.

What the Critics Say

While a low-fat, high-carbohydrate diet is widely considered healthy, some experts worry that a strict macrobiotic diet does not have enough variety, especially for children and pregnant women. Iron, calcium and some vitamins are particular concerns on such a limited diet. Extremely restrictive versions that rely almost solely on grains could be dangerously low in protein and other nutrients for anyone.

Research is being conducted to determine the effect of macrobiotic food on the progress of some cancers. However, even some of those who support the diet and its avoidance of processed foods and saturated fats caution that there is so far no good evidence that any diet alone can cure disease.

Nutrition and Diet

Mediterranean Diet

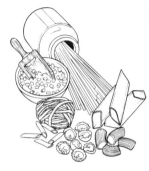

The populations of 15 countries on three different continents live near the Mediterranean Sea, and despite variations from culture to culture, they share a remarkably similar traditional diet. Staples include grains, potatoes, pasta, pulses, vegetables, garlic and olive oil. Sweets and most animal products are limited. Some fish is consumed, mostly of the oily varieties, such as mullet and tuna.

What It's Good For

Quantities of complex carbohydrates and fresh vegetables align this diet with the Food Guide Pyramid's recommendations.

- **Heart disease:** The Mediterranean diet is quite high in fat, but it is mostly monounsaturated fat from olive oil, which has been shown to reduce the 'bad' kind of cholesterol (low-density lipoprotein, or LDL) without lowering the amount of 'good' cholesterol (high-density lipoprotein, or HDL) in the body—and so may help protect against heart disease.

  Omega-3 fatty acids present in oily fish seem to help lower blood cholesterol levels, and the vitamins and beta carotene present in brightly coloured vegetables can protect the body against heart disease. Large amounts of garlic may be effective in lowering blood pressure.

  Mediterranean cultures traditionally consume red wine with meals. Some studies indicate that moderate consumption of red wine may help reduce the risk of heart disease for certain individuals.

- **Diabetes:** A high level of monounsaturated fats in the diet has been shown to help control blood sugar levels in the adult-onset type of diabetes.

- **Cancer:** The diet's emphasis on complex carbohydrates may help protect against bowel cancer.

Preparations/Techniques

Specifics of the Mediterranean diet vary from culture to culture, and recipes are widely available. Two simple ways to get some of the benefits of this diet are to substitute olive oil for other fats, and to add more vegetables and garlic to your meals.

What the Critics Say

Olive oil is not a cure-all; you still must ensure enough variety in your diet to get all the nutrients you need.

CONTINUED

Nutrition and Diet CONTINUED

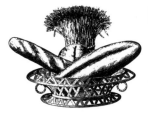

Vegetarian Diet

Many cultures have a longstanding tradition of avoiding the consumption of some or all animal products. The several forms of vegetarianism are among the most popular alternatives to the standard diet today. Some people believe that humans are physically better suited to digesting grains, beans, vegetables and fruits than meat and other animal products; others avoid meat for philosophical or ecological reasons. In general, vegetarians enjoy a diet lower in fat and higher in complex carbohydrates than one with a lot of red meat and other animal products

What It's Good For

Cutting your fat intake from animal products can be beneficial in many ways.
- **Heart disease:** Lower amounts of saturated fats and higher intake of polyunsaturated fats and fibre may help lower blood pressure and prevent heart disease.
- **Digestive disorders:** Higher consumption of fibre-rich foods may help vegetarians avoid diverticular disease and bowel cancer.

Preparations/Techniques

Vegans eat no animal foods at all. Lactovegetarians consume dairy products but no eggs or meat. Lacto-ovo-vegetarians eat eggs and milk products but no meat. Others exclude only red meat; some also abstain from either poultry or fish.

Take care to get enough variety to ensure proper nutrition. Protein is available from beans, grains and some vegetables. Vitamin B_{12} is a special worry on a vegetarian diet because there is no good plant source—supplements are necessary. Other micronutrients to be concerned about are vitamin D (available from egg yolks, fortified milk, or adequate sunshine); calcium (milk, fortified soya bean milk and dark green vegetables except spinach and chard); riboflavin (dark green vegetables, pulses and whole grains); and iron (use iron cookware, eat soya beans and ensure a plentiful intake of foods containing ascorbic acid to boost absorption of iron).

What the Critics Say

Nutrition experts generally warn pregnant or lactating women to be very careful to assure adequate nutrition on this diet. Also, there is concern for children; rapid growth requires plenty of protein and adequate amounts of several micronutrients that can be in short supply in a totally vegetarian diet. A dietitian or nutritionist can help safeguard your well-being. For most adults who make wise food choices, vegetarianism can supply a healthy diet. ■

The 32 Most Common Vitamins and Minerals

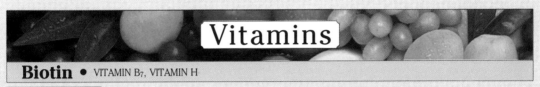

Vitamins

Biotin • VITAMIN B₇, VITAMIN H

RDA:
150 mcg

Along with other B vitamins, biotin helps convert food to energy and is required for the synthesis of carbohydrates, proteins and fatty acids. Biotin is especially important for maintaining the health of hair, skin and nails.

Among the types of food that are good dietary sources of biotin are cheese, kidneys, salmon, soya beans, sunflower seeds, nuts, broccoli and sweet potatoes. Biotin deficiency is rare, and supplements are unnecessary. People can become biotin deficient through long-term use of antibiotics or by regularly eating raw egg whites, which contain avidin, a protein that blocks the body's absorption of biotin.

Because breast milk contains little biotin, infants who are breast-fed can suffer biotin deficiency, although this is uncommon. Signs of biotin deficiency include a scaly, oily skin rash; hair loss; nausea; vomiting; muscle pain; loss of appetite; a red, inflamed tongue; and fatigue. Research has not revealed a toxic level for biotin. ■

Folic Acid • VITAMIN B₉, FOLACIN, FOLATE

RDA:
200 mcg

Healthy hair, skin, nails, nerves, mucous membranes and blood all depend on folic acid. A critical component of RNA and DNA—the genetic material that controls the growth and repair of all cells—folic acid supports immune function and may help deter atherosclerosis as well as some cancers of the mucous membranes.

Sources of folic acid include liver, kidneys, avocado pears, beans, beetroot, celery, eggs, fish, green leafy vegetables, nuts, seeds, peas, orange juice and vitamin-fortified breakfast cereals. A healthy diet should provide adequate folic acid, but the need increases during pregnancy, with injury, with some diseases—especially cancer—and with long-term use of drugs such as aspirin and oral contraceptives. Supplements taken three months before and during pregnancy may help deter the birth defects spina bifida and cleft palate. For this reason, some experts now recommend that women of childbearing age consume 400 mcg daily. It may also help prevent heart disease, and there is some evidence that it may prevent Alzheimer's disease. High doses of folic acid are not toxic but may mask the symptoms of vitamin B₁₂ deficiency. Therefore, it's best to increase folic acid intake through diet or a multivitamin that contains a low dose of folic acid

Extreme vitamin B₉ deficiency may cause megaloblastic anaemia, a disease characterized by red blood cells that are too few in number and malformed. Symptoms include pallor; fatigue; loss of appetite; insomnia; diarrhoea; and a red, inflamed tongue. Those who are most susceptible to folic acid deficiency include alcoholics, people with gastrointestinal diseases, adolescents who subsist mainly on junk food, women taking oral contraceptives and pregnant women who are not taking supplements. ■

Niacin • VITAMIN B₃, NICOTINIC ACID

RDA:
18 mg

Niacin contributes to more than 50 vital bodily processes: It helps convert food into energy; build red blood cells; synthesize hormones, steroids, and fatty acids; maintain the skin, nerves and blood vessels; support the gastrointestinal tract; stabilize mental health; and detoxify certain drugs and chemicals in the body. In addition, it helps insulin regulate blood sugar levels. Niacin is also a powerful drug, capable of lowering blood cholesterol and triglycerides, dilating blood vessels to improve circulation, and alleviating depression, insomnia, and hyperactivity.

Foods rich in niacin include liver, poultry, lean meats, fish, nuts, peanut butter and enriched flour. If you get enough protein, you are probably getting enough nicotinic acid. If adequate vitamin B₆ is present, the body can also produce niacin from the amino acid tryptophan, found in milk, eggs, and cheese. Signs of deficiency include indigestion, diarrhoea, muscle weakness, appetite loss, dermatitis made

CONTINUED

worse by sunlight, mouth sores, an inflamed tongue, headaches, irritability, anxiety and depression. Pregnant or breastfeeding women, the elderly, alcoholics, and people with hyperthyroidism are most likely to be niacin deficient. Extreme deficiency results in pellagra, characterized by diarrhoea, dermatitis and mental illness. It was common until the discovery that niacin was a cure; the disease is now virtually nonexistent in the West thanks to enriched flour and other foods. Multivitamin supplements can raise nicotinic acid levels safely. The nutrient is toxic in high amounts, so avoid megadoses. Nausea, which often prevents further intake, is the first symptom; continued overuse may cause a rash, itchy skin and liver damage. ∎

Vitamin A • BETA CAROTENE, RETINOL, RETINENE, RETINOIC ACID, RETINYL PALMITATE

RDA:
800 mcg

The first vitamin ever discovered, vitamin A is essential for good vision—especially in dim light—and for healthy skin, hair and mucous membranes of the nose, throat, respiratory system and digestive system. This vitamin is also necessary for the proper development of bones and teeth. It stimulates wound healing and is used to treat some skin disorders. Beta carotene, the precursor to vitamin A, is a carotenoid, a type of pigment found in plants. Your skin stores beta carotene and your body metabolizes it to produce vitamin A as needed. Excess beta carotene, along with other carotenoids, acts as an antioxidant and supports immune function, so it increases your resistance to infection; it may help prevent vision problems such as night blindness and some cancers (although megadoses have been implicated in causing others). Beta carotene may also help lower cholesterol levels and reduce the risk of heart disease.

Vitamin A is present in orange and yellow vegetables and fruits; dark green leafy vegetables such as mustard greens and kale; whole milk, cream and butter; and organ meats. Because it is fat soluble, vitamin A is stored in the body for a long time, and supplements are generally not recommended. Too much vitamin A can cause headaches, vision problems, nausea, vomiting, dry and flaking skin, or an enlarged liver or spleen. ∎

Vitamin B Complex

RDA:
See individual
vitamin entries

As its name implies, vitamin B complex is a combination, or mixture, of eight essential vitamins. Although each is chemically distinct, the B vitamins coexist in many of the same foods and often work together to bolster metabolism, maintain healthy skin and muscle tone, enhance immune and nervous system function and promote cell growth and division—including that of the red blood cells that help prevent anaemia.

Foods rich in B-complex vitamins include liver and other organ meats, fish, poultry, brewer's yeast, eggs, beans and peas, dark green leafy vegetables, whole-grain cereals, and dairy products. B vitamins, which are water soluble, are dispersed throughout the body and must be replenished daily; any excess is excreted in urine. People susceptible to vitamin B deficiency include pregnant women, nursing mothers, vegetarians, alcoholics, 'sugarholics', the elderly and people who have malabsorption conditions or who take certain antibiotics over a long period of time; the symptoms include oily and scaly skin, upset stomach, headaches, anxiety, moodiness and heart arrhythmias. A deficiency of one B vitamin usually means that intake of all B vitamins is low. If your doctor suggests you need more B vitamins, take a daily multivitamin or B-complex supplement rather than individual B-vitamin supplements. Most B vitamins are nontoxic unless taken in excessively large amounts. ∎

Thiamine • VITAMIN B₁

RDA:
1.4 mg

Thiamine, sometimes called the energy vitamin because it is needed to metabolize carbohydrates, fats, and proteins, helps convert excess glucose into stored fat. It also ensures proper nerve impulse transmission and contributes to maintaining normal appetite, muscle tone, and mental health. In the 1930s thiamine was discovered to be the cure for the crippling and potentially fatal disease beriberi. Now that rice, flour and bread are generally enriched with thiamine, beriberi is relatively rare.

A diet that regularly includes lean pork, milk, whole grains, peas, beans, peanuts or soya beans generally provides enough thiamine. Athletes, laborers, pregnant women and others who burn lots of energy may require more than the RDA of thiamine. Mild deficiency may cause fatigue, loss of appetite, nausea, moodiness, confusion, anae-mia and possibly heart arrhythmias. Alcohol suppresses thiamine absorption; for this reason and because of typically poor diets, alcoholics are likely to be deficient in thiamine and other nutrients. To increase thiamine levels, try changing your diet or taking a multivitamin rather than thiamine supplements. Large doses up to 100 mg of thiamine may alleviate itching from insect bites; otherwise, megasupplements are not known to be either harmful or helpful. ∎

Riboflavin • VITAMIN B$_2$

RDA:
1.6 mg

Like other members of the vitamin B complex, riboflavin helps produce energy from carbohydrates, fats and proteins. Riboflavin also promotes healthy skin, hair, nails, and mucous membranes; aids the production of red blood cells, corticosteroids, and thyroid hormones; and is required for the proper function of the nerves, eyes and adrenal glands. It is often used to treat acne, anaemia, cataracts and depression.

A well-balanced diet provides most people with adequate riboflavin, although athletes and others who need a great deal of energy may require more than the RDA. Lean organ meats, enriched bread and flour, cheese, yoghurt, eggs, almonds, soya bean products such as tofu, and green leafy vegetables—especially broccoli—are good sources. Store these foods in the dark because riboflavin breaks down in sunlight. Alcoholics and elderly people are susceptible to riboflavin deficiency: The signs include oily, scaly skin rash; sores, especially on the lips and corners of the mouth; a swollen, red, painful tongue; sensitivity to light; and burning or red, itchy eyes. Although vitamin B$_2$ supplements are available, they provide far more riboflavin than anyone needs. Diet changes are better, or take a multivitamin supplement. It is best to take the supplements with food, which increases their absorption tremendously compared with tablets alone. ∎

Pantothenic acid • VITAMIN B$_5$

RDA:
6 mg

The Greek term *pan* in *pantothenic acid* means 'everywhere', indicating this vitamin's abundance. Along with other B vitamins, pantothenic acid is required for converting food to energy; building red blood cells; making bile; and synthesizing fats, adrenal gland steroids, antibodies and acetylcholine and other neurotransmitters—chemicals that permit nerve transmission. Pantothenic acid in dexpanthenol lotions and creams relieves the pain of burns, cuts and abrasions; reduces skin inflammation; and speeds the healing of wounds.

Panthothenic acid is abundant in organ meats, dark turkey meat, salmon, wheat bran, brewer's yeast, brown rice, lentils, nuts, beans, sweetcorn, peas, sweet potatoes and eggs. Excess pantothenic acid may cause diarrhoea. A deficiency in this vitamin does not seem to occur naturally in humans and is likely only with extreme starvation. A pantothenic acid supplement, calcium pantothenate, is available. ∎

Vitamin B$_6$ • PYRIDOXINE

RDA:
2 mg

Vitamin B$_6$ encompasses a family of compounds that includes pyridoxine, pyridoxamine and pyridoxal. This vitamin supports immune function, transmission of nerve impulses (especially in the brain), energy metabolism and synthesis of red blood cells. Prescribed as a drug, it can sometimes alleviate carpal tunnel syndrome, infant seizures and PMS.

A healthy diet provides enough vitamin B$_6$ for most people. Brown rice, lean meats, poultry, fish, bananas, avocado pears, whole grains, sweetcorn and nuts are rich in vitamin B$_6$. People most likely to be at risk for vitamin B$_6$ deficiency include anyone with a malabsorption problem such as lactose intolerance or coeliac disease; diabetic or elderly people; and women who are pregnant, nursing, or taking

CONTINUED

oral contraceptives. Severe deficiency is rare. Mild deficiency may cause acne and inflamed skin, insomnia, muscle weakness, nausea, irritability, depression and fatigue. A daily multivitamin supplement is usually recommended to boost low vitamin B_6 levels. Taking too much or too little vitamin B_6 can impair nerve function and mental health. If high levels (2,000–5,000 mg) are taken for several months, vitamin B_6 can become habit forming and may induce sleepiness as well as tingling, numb hands and feet. These symptoms will most likely disappear when the vitamin B_6 intake is reduced, and there is usually no permanent damage. ■

Vitamin B_{12} • COBALAMIN

RDA:
1 mcg

The largest and most complex family of the B vitamins, Vitamin B_{12} includes several chemical compounds known as cobalamins. Cyanocobalamin, the stablest form, is the one most likely to be found in supplements. Like other B vitamins, B_{12} is important for converting fats, carbohydrates and protein into energy, and assisting in the synthesis of red blood cells. It is critical for producing the genetic materials RNA and DNA, as well as myelin, a fatty substance that forms a protective sheath around nerves. Unlike other B vitamins, vitamin B_{12} needs several hours to be absorbed in the digestive tract. Excess vitamin B_{12} is excreted in urine, even though a backup supply can be stored for several years in the liver.

Vitamin B_{12} is not produced by plants but is supplied through animal products such as organ meats, fish, eggs and dairy products. Dietary deficiency is uncommon and is usually limited to alcoholics, strict vegetarians and pregnant or nursing women—who should take supplements. More often, deficiency stems from an inability to absorb the vitamin, a problem that may occur for years before symptoms show; it tends to affect the elderly, those who have had stomach surgery or people who have a disease of malabsorption, such as colitis.

Lack of calcium, vitamin B_6 or iron may also interfere with the normal absorption of B_{12}. Signs of vitamin B_{12} deficiency include a sore tongue, weakness, weight loss, body odour, back pains and tingling arms and legs. Severe deficiency leads to pernicious anaemia, causing fatigue, a tendency to bleed, lemon yellow pallor, abdominal pain, stiff arms and legs, irritability and depression.

Without treatment, pernicious anaemia can lead to permanent nerve damage and possibly death; the disease can be controlled, although not cured, with regular B_{12} injections. Vitamin B_{12} is considered non-toxic, even when taken at several times the RDA. ■

Vitamin C • ASCORBIC ACID

RDA:
60 mg

Vitamin C is well known for its ability to prevent and treat scurvy, a disease that causes swollen and bleeding gums, aching bones and muscles and, in some cases, even death. It is also essential to the healing of wounds, burns, bruises and broken bones because collagen, the substance that constitutes the body's connective tissue, depends on vitamin C for its production. As a powerful anti-oxidant and immune system booster, vitamin C may alleviate the pain of rheumatoid arthritis, protect against atherosclerosis and heart disease, and help prevent some forms of cancer; and has the reputed potential capacity (yet unproved) to prevent the common cold. More than the RDA may be needed under conditions of physical or emotional stress.

Sources of vitamin C include citrus fruits, rose hips, bell peppers, strawberries, broccoli, melons, tomatoes and leafy greens. Vitamin C breaks down faster than any other vitamin, so it is best to eat fruits and vegetables when fresh and to cook them minimally or not at all. Slight vitamin C deficiency is rather common, although severe deficiencies are rare in the West today. Symptoms of deficiency include weight loss, fatigue, bleeding gums, easy bruising, reduced resistance to colds and other infections and slow healing of wounds and fractures.

Because it is water soluble, excess vitamin C is excreted in the urine, so large amounts of it may usually be taken without fear of toxicity. Doses larger than 1,000 mg a day have been suggested for preventing cancer, infections such as the common cold and other ailments. In some people, large doses may induce such side effects as nausea, diarrhoea, reduced selenium and copper absorption, excessive iron absorption, increased kidney stone formation and a false-positive reaction to diabetes tests. ■

The 32 Most Common Vitamins and Minerals

Vitamin D • CHOLECALCIFEROL, ERGOCALCIFEROL

RDA:
5 mcg

Vitamin D not only promotes healthy bones and teeth by regulating the absorption and balance of calcium and phosphorus, but also fosters normal muscle contraction and nerve function. Vitamin D prevents rickets, a disease of calcium-deprived bone that results in bowlegs, knock-knees and other bone defects. Vitamin D supplements may help treat psoriasis and slow or even reverse some cancers, such as myeloid leukaemia.

Fatty fish such as herring, salmon and tuna, followed by dairy products, are the richest natural sources of this nutrient. Few other foods naturally contain vitamin D, but 10 minutes in midday summer sun enables the body to produce about 200 IU of it. Milk, breakfast cereals and infant formulas are fortified with vitamin D. In adults, vitamin D deficiency can cause nervousness and diarrhoea, insomnia, muscle twitches and bone weakening, and it may worsen osteoporosis. Too much vitamin D raises the calcium level in the blood, which in turn may induce headaches, nausea, loss of appetite, excessive thirst, muscle weakness and even heart, liver, or kidney damage as calcium deposits accumulate in soft tissue. Vitamin D is fat soluble; excess amounts of it are stored in the body. Because of its potentially toxic effects, vitamin D should not be taken in supplements of more than 400 IU daily unless prescribed by a doctor. ■

Vitamin E

RDA:
10 mg

Vitamin E encompasses a family of compounds called tocopherols, of which alpha-tocopherol is the most common. It is required for proper function of the immune system, endocrine system, and sex glands. As a potent anti-oxidant, it prevents unstable molecules known as free radicals from damaging cells and tissues. In this capacity, vitamin E deters atherosclerosis, accelerates wound healing, protects lung tissue from inhaled pollutants and may reduce risk of heart disease and prevent premature ageing of skin. Researchers suspect that vitamin E has other beneficial effects ranging from preventing cancer and cataracts to alleviating rheumatoid arthritis and a skin disorder associated with lupus.

Most people get enough vitamin E through their diet and don't need supplements. Vegetable oils, nuts, dark green leafy vegetables, organ meats, seafood, eggs and avocado pears are rich food sources. Symptoms of vitamin E deficiency, such as fluid retention and haemolytic anaemia, are rare in adults but are sometimes seen in premature infants. Because of its many suggested therapeutic roles, vitamin E is popular as an oral supplement and an ingredient of skin-care products. Although it is fat soluble, vitamin E is considered non-toxic because it does no harm except in extremely high doses. ■

Vitamin K • MENADIONE, PHYTONADIONE

RDA:
Not established

Vitamin K is needed in a small but critical amount to form certain proteins essential mainly for blood clotting but also for kidney function and bone metabolism. Vitamin K exists in two natural forms that require some dietary fat for absorption.

Bacteria living in the intestines produce about half the body's needs; the rest comes from diet. Good food sources include spinach, cabbage, broccoli, turnip greens or other leafy vegetables; beef liver; green tea; cheese; and oats. Vitamin K deficiency is extremely rare in adults but may occur in newborns until their intestinal bacteria begin producing the vitamin. To enhance blood-clotting ability in a newborn, the mother may take vitamin K supplements before delivery, and infants usually receive them after birth. Otherwise, supplements are neither necessary nor recommended. Megadoses higher than 500 mcg can be toxic or cause an allergic reaction and must be prescribed by a doctor. Large doses of vitamin E may interfere with vitamin K's blood-clotting effects. ■

CONTINUED

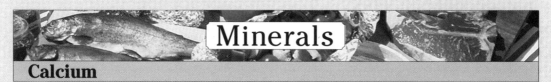

Minerals

Calcium

RDA:
800 mg

Calcium, the most abundant mineral in the body, is essential for the growth and maintenance of bones and teeth. It enables muscles, including the heart, to contract; it is essential for normal blood clotting, proper nerve-impulse transmission and connective tissue maintenance. It helps keep blood pressure normal and may reduce the risk of heart disease; taken with vitamin D, it may help lessen the risk of bowel cancer. It helps prevent rickets in children and osteoporosis in adults.

Good sources include dairy products, dark green leafy vegetables, sardines, salmon and almonds. Calcium is needed in varying amounts by different people. Too much calcium can lead to constipation and to calcium deposits in soft tissue, causing damage to the heart, liver or kidneys. For calcium to be properly absorbed, the body must have sufficient levels of vitamin D and of hydrochloric acid in the stomach and a balance of other minerals, including magnesium and phosphorus. A sedentary lifestyle and consuming too much alcohol, dietary fibre and fat can interfere with calcium absorption; too much protein and caffeine results in calcium being excreted in urine. Supplemental calcium is available in many forms; the form that is best absorbed by the body is calcium citrate-malate. ∎

Chloride

RDA:
Not established

A natural salt of the mineral chlorine, chloride works with sodium and potassium to help maintain the proper distribution and pH of all bodily fluids and to encourage healthy nerve and muscle function. Independently, chloride contributes to digestion and waste elimination. It is a key component of hydrochloric acid, one of the gastric juices that digest food.

A diet of unprocessed natural foods provides more than enough chloride for human health. Just a pinch of table salt contains about 250 mg, about one-third of the amount many nutritionists recommend. Chloride deficiency is extremely rare and is usually due to illness. Excessive vomiting can reduce the stomach's chloride level, upsetting its pH balance and causing sweating, diarrhoea, loss of appetite, slow and shallow breathing, listlessness, and muscle cramps. Although toxic in large amounts, excess chloride is excreted in urine, preventing potentially dangerous accumulation. ∎

Chromium

RDA:
Not established

As a component of a natural substance called glucose tolerance factor, chromium works with insulin to regulate the body's use of sugar and is essential to fatty-acid metabolism. Its contribution to metabolism makes chromium a helpful supplement in weight-loss programmes. Additional evidence suggests that chromium may help deter atherosclerosis and reduce the risk of cardiovascular disease. Inadequate chromium can result in alcohol intolerance, elevate blood sugar levels, and possibly induce diabetes-like symptoms such as tingling in the extremities and reduced muscle coordination.

Trace amounts of chromium are found in many foods, including brewer's yeast, liver, lean meats, poultry, treacle, whole grains, eggs and cheese. Chromium is not absorbed well, so the body must take in far more than it actually uses. Most people do not get enough dietary chromium, and some may benefit from a multi-nutrient supplement, such as chromium citrate or chromium picolinate. Supplemental chromium may be used to treat some cases of adult-onset diabetes, to reduce insulin requirements of some diabetic children, and to relieve symptoms of hypoglycaemia. Taken regularly in supplements greater than 1,000 mcg, however, chromium inhibits insulin's activity and can be toxic. ∎

The 32 Most Common Vitamins and Minerals

Cobalt

RDA:
Not established

The mineral cobalt is a constituent of cobalamin (vitamin B_{12}). Cobalt helps form red blood cells and maintain nerve tissue. Consuming large amounts of inorganic cobalt stimulates growth of the thyroid gland and may lead to the overproduction of red blood cells, a disorder known as polycythaemia.

To be biologically useful, cobalt must be obtained from foods such as liver, kidneys, milk, oysters, clams or sea vegetables, or from vitamin B_{12} supplements. Inorganic cobalt has no nutritional value but is sometimes added to lager as an anti-foaming agent. ∎

Copper

RDA:
Not established

Copper is indispensable to human health. Its many functions include the following: helping to form haemoglobin in the blood; facilitating the absorption and use of iron so that red blood cells can transport oxygen to tissues; assisting in the regulation of blood pressure and heart rate; strengthening blood vessels, bones, tendons and nerves; promoting fertility; and ensuring normal skin and hair pigmentation. Some evidence suggests that copper helps prevent cardiovascular problems such as high blood pressure and heart arrhythmias and that it may help treat arthritis and scoliosis. Copper may also protect tissue from damage by free radicals, support the body's immune function and contribute to preventing cancer.

Most adults get enough copper from a normal, varied diet. Seafood and organ meats are the richest sources; treacle, nuts, seeds, green vegetables, black pepper, cocoa and water passed through copper pipes also contain significant quantities. Supplemental copper should be taken only on a doctor's advice. Common supplemental forms are copper aspartate, copper citrate and copper picolinate. Excess calcium and zinc will interfere with copper absorption, but a true copper deficiency is rare and tends to be limited to people either with certain inherited diseases that inhibit copper absorption, such as albinism, or with acquired malabsorption ailments, such as Crohn's disease and coeliac disease. The deficiency may also occur in infants who are not breast-fed and in some premature babies. Symptoms of copper deficiency include brittle, discoloured hair; skeletal defects; anaemia; high blood pressure; heart arrhythmias; and infertility. Taking more than 10 mg of copper daily can bring on nausea, vomiting, muscle pain and stomach aches. Women who are pregnant or taking birth-control pills are susceptible to excess blood levels of copper. Some research suggests that high levels of copper and iron may play a role in hyperactivity and autism. ∎

Fluoride

RDA:
Not established

Fluoride, a natural form of the mineral fluorine, is required for healthy teeth and bones. It helps form the tough enamel that protects the teeth from decay, and increases bone strength and stability. Since the 1950s, some cities have added fluoride to municipal drinking water at a ratio of about 1 part per million (ppm), or 1 mg per litre. Many believe this practice is responsible for the sharp decline in tooth decay that dentists have since observed. Fluoride's decay-reducing effects are strongest if children are exposed to the mineral while their teeth are forming. Fluoride toothpaste is helpful, but it is not nearly as effective as regularly ingested fluoride.

Fluoridated water provides most individuals with at least 1 mg of fluoride per day; other dietary sources are dried seaweed, seafood—especially sardines and salmon—cheese, meat and tea. Nursing babies and children who do not regularly drink fluoridated water should be given supplements, but only as prescribed by a dentist or doctor, because excess fluoride can have adverse effects: At levels of 2 ppm to 8 ppm, the teeth may soften and discolour; at over 8 ppm, fluoride toxicity can depress growth, harden ligaments and tendons, make bones brittle and induce degeneration of major body systems; 50 ppm may cause fatal poisoning. The low fluoride levels in fluoridated drinking water, however, pose no harmful effects to health. ∎

CONTINUED

The 32 Most Common Vitamins and Minerals

Iodine

RDA:
150 mcg

Iodine was one of the first minerals recognized as essential to human health. For centuries, it has been known to prevent and treat goitre—enlargement of the thyroid gland. As part of several thyroid hormones, iodine strongly influences nutrient metabolism; nerve and muscle function; skin, hair, tooth and nail condition; and physical and mental development. Iodine may also help convert beta carotene into vitamin A.

Kelp, seafood and vegetables grown in iodine-rich soils are good sources of this mineral. Some salt is iodized, supplying sufficient iodine in a regular diet. Supplements are usually unnecessary, but pregnant women should take in enough iodine for themselves and their babies to prevent potential mental retardation or cretinism, a form of dwarfism in infants. Iodine deficiency is now uncommon; besides goitre, its effects include weight gain, hair loss, listlessness, insomnia and some forms of mental retardation. Most excess iodine is excreted, but extremely high intake may cause nervousness, hyperactivity, headache, rashes, a metallic taste in the mouth, and goitre—in this case, due to thyroid hyperactivity. ■

Iron

RDA:
14 mg

Iron is found in haemoglobin, the protein in red blood cells that transports oxygen from the lungs to body tissues. It is also a component of myoglobin, a protein that provides extra fuel to muscles during exertion.

Dietary iron exists in two forms: haem iron, found in red meat, chicken, seafood, and other animal products; and non-haem iron, found in dark green vegetables, whole grains, nuts, dried fruit and other plant foods. Many flour-based food products are fortified with iron. Haem iron is easier to absorb, but eating foods containing non-haem iron along with foods that have haem iron or vitamin C will maximize iron absorption.

Coffee, tea, soya-based foods, antacids and tetracycline inhibit iron absorption, as do excessive amounts of calcium, zinc and manganese. Lack of iron deprives body tissues of oxygen and may cause iron-deficiency anaemia; warning signs include fatigue, paleness, dizziness, sensitivity to cold, listlessness, irritability, poor concentration and heart palpitations. Because iron strengthens immune function, iron deficiency also may increase susceptibility to infection. Women need more iron before menopause than after, because menstruation causes iron loss each month. People who have special iron intake needs include menstruating or pregnant women, children under two years of age, vegetarians, anyone with bleeding conditions such as haemorrhoids or bleeding stomach ulcers, and anyone taking the medications listed above.

On a doctor's recommendation, adults can augment their iron intake by means of a multi-nutrient supplement; straight iron supplements should be taken only under a doctor's supervision. Excess iron inhibits absorption of phosphorus, interferes with immune function and may increase your risk of developing cancer, cirrhosis or heart attack. Symptoms of iron toxicity include diarrhoea, vomiting, headache, dizziness, fatigue, stomach cramps and weak pulse. Though uncommon, severe iron poisoning can result in coma, heart failure and death. Children should never be given adult iron supplements, which can easily poison them. If your doctor recommends an iron supplement for your child, make sure it is a specific, child-formulated variety. ■

Magnesium

RDA:
300 mg

Magnesium contributes to health in many ways. Along with calcium and phosphorus, it is a main constituent of bone. A proper balance of calcium and magnesium is essential for healthy bones and teeth, reduces the risk of developing osteoporosis and may minimize the effects of existing osteoporosis. Calcium and magnesium also help regulate muscle activity. While calcium stimulates contraction, magnesium induces relaxation. Magnesium is essential for metabolism—converting food to energy—and for building proteins. Adequate blood levels of magnesium protect the body from cardiovascular disease, heart arrhythmias and, possibly, stroke due to blood clotting in the brain.

On average, people get enough (or nearly enough)

The 32 Most Common Vitamins and Minerals

magnesium in their diet. Fish, green leafy vegetables, milk, nuts, seeds and whole grains are good sources. Many over-the-counter antacids, laxatives and analgesics contain magnesium, but these medications should not be used as magnesium supplements. A multi-nutrient supplement is a relatively safe way to augment your magnesium intake. Take specific magnesium supplements only under a doctor's supervision. Of the supplemental forms, magnesium citrate-malate is the easiest to absorb, while magnesium glycinate is the least likely to cause diarrhoea at high doses.

The body's need for magnesium increases with stress or illness. Administered as a supplement, magnesium may successfully treat insomnia, muscle cramps, premenstrual syndrome and cardiovascular problems including high blood pressure, angina due to coronary artery spasm, and leg pain and cramping due to insufficient blood flow. Studies indicate that giving magnesium immediately to a heart attack patient greatly increases the chance of survival.

The body processes magnesium efficiently; the kidneys conserve it as needed and excrete any excess, so both severe deficiency and toxicity are rare. These conditions are dangerous when they do occur, however. Magnesium deficiency may cause nausea, listlessness, muscle weakness, tremor, disorientation and heart palpitations. Toxicity can induce diarrhoea, fatigue, muscle weakness and, in extreme cases, severely depressed heart rate and blood pressure, shallow breathing, loss of reflexes, coma and possibly death. People who abuse laxatives or experience kidney failure are the most vulnerable to magnesium poisoning. ∎

Manganese

RDA:
Not established

Manganese is essential for the proper formation and maintenance of bone, cartilage and connective tissue; it contributes to the synthesis of proteins and genetic material; it helps produce energy from foods; it acts as an anti-oxidant; and it assists in normal blood clotting.

Most people get enough manganese through their diet alone; for example, a breakfast consisting of orange juice, a 1-oz (30 g) serving of bran cereal and a banana provides just over 2.5 mg of manganese. Other food sources include brown rice, nuts, seeds, wheat germ, beans, whole grains, peas and strawberries. Manganese citrate, a supplement, may help repair damaged tendons and ligaments. Excess dietary manganese is not considered toxic, and manganese deficiency is extremely rare. ∎

Molybdenum

RDA:
Not established

The obscure mineral molybdenum is an enzyme component. It helps generate energy, process waste for excretion, mobilize stored iron for the body's use and detoxify sulphites—chemicals used as food preservatives. As such, molybdenum is essential to normal development, particularly of the nervous system. It is also a component of tooth enamel and may help prevent tooth decay.

Molybdenum is present in peas, beans, cereals, pasta, leafy vegetables, yeast, milk and organ meats. People generally get enough through diet; deficiency is virtually non-existent. Toxicity is also rare. Molybdenum is available in supplement form as molybdenum picolinate; however, prolonged intake of more than 10 mg daily can cause gout-like symptoms such as joint pain and swelling. ∎

Phosphorus

RDA:
800 mg

Phosphorus is the second most plentiful mineral in the body and is found in every cell. Like calcium, phosphorus is essential for bone formation and maintenance; more than 75 per cent of the body's phosphorus is contained in bones and teeth. Phosphorus stimulates muscle contraction and contributes to tissue growth and repair, energy production, nerve-impulse transmission and heart and kidney function.

Phosphorus exists to some degree in nearly all foods, especially meats, poultry, eggs, fish, nuts, dairy products, whole grains and soft drinks. Deficiency is rare—most people take in far more phosphorus than they need—but may

CONTINUED

be induced by long-term use of antacids or anticonvulsant drugs that contain aluminum hydroxide. Symptoms of phosphorus deficiency include general weakness, loss of appetite, bone pain and increased susceptibility to bone fracture. Excess phosphorus in the bloodstream promotes calcium loss, which may weaken bones. Extreme phosphorus toxicity is rare, except in the event of kidney disease. ∎

Potassium

RDA:
Not established

Potassium is the third most abundant mineral in the body. It works closely with sodium and chloride to maintain fluid distribution and pH balance and to augment nerve-impulse transmission, muscle contraction and regulation of heartbeat and blood pressure. It is also required for protein synthesis, carbohydrate metabolism and insulin secretion by the pancreas. Studies suggest that people who regularly eat potassium-rich foods are less likely to develop atherosclerosis, heart disease and high blood pressure, or to die of a stroke.

Dietary sources include lean meats, raw vegetables, fruits—especially citrus fruits, bananas and avocado pears—and potatoes. Many people may get only marginal amounts of potassium, but supplements, such as potassium aspartate, are best taken only under a doctor's guidance. Marginal potassium deficiency causes no symptoms but may increase the risk of developing high blood pressure or aggravate existing heart disease. More severe deficiency can result in nausea, diarrhoea, muscle cramps and muscle weakness, poor reflexes, poor concentration, heart arrhythmias and, rarely, death due to heart failure. Acute potassium toxicity may have similar effects, including possible heart failure. However, acute toxicity is rarely linked to diet and tends to occur only in the event of kidney failure. ∎

Selenium

RDA:
Not established

An anti-oxidant, selenium protects cells and tissues from damage wrought by free radicals. Because its anti-oxidant effects complement those of vitamin E, the two are said to potentiate, or reinforce, each other. Selenium also supports immune function and neutralizes certain poisonous substances such as cadmium, mercury and arsenic that may be ingested or inhaled. Although its full therapeutic value is unknown, adequate selenium levels may help combat arthritis, deter heart disease and prevent cancer.

Whole grains, asparagus, garlic, eggs and mushrooms are typically good sources, as are lean meats and seafood. Very little selenium is required for good health, and most people get adequate amounts through diet alone. High-dose supplements such as selenium citrate and selenium picolinate should be taken only if prescribed by a doctor. Selenium can be toxic in extremely high doses, causing hair loss, nail problems, accelerated tooth decay and swelling of the fingers, among other symptoms. Some multi-nutrients contain selenium, but always in small, safe amounts. Selenium-containing shampoo is excellent against dandruff. ∎

Sodium

RDA:
Not established

All bodily fluids—including blood, tears and perspiration—contain the mineral sodium. Together with potassium and chloride, sodium maintains fluid distribution and pH balance; with potassium, sodium also helps control muscle contraction and nerve function.

Most of the sodium in the Western diet is from table salt. Among many other sources are processed foods, soft drinks, meats, shellfish, condiments, snack foods, food additives and over-the-counter laxatives. We generally consume far too much sodium. A single teaspoon of salt contains 2,000 mg—four times the daily minimum many nutritionists recommend—but average daily consumption is usually much more than this.

Keeping sodium intake within reasonable limits is critical to maintaining long-term health. When sodium levels are persistently elevated, the body loses potassium and retains water, making blood pressure rise. Adopting a low-sodium

The 32 Most Common Vitamins and Minerals

diet can reduce high blood pressure and correct a potassium deficiency. Over-exertion, particularly in the hot sun, can induce temporary sodium deficiency, which is characterized by nausea, dehydration, muscle cramps and other symptoms of heatstroke and exhaustion. Drinking several glasses of water with a pinch of salt added replaces the sodium and eases the symptoms. ■

Sulphur

RDA:
Not established

Accounting for some 10 per cent of the body's mineral content, sulphur is part of every cell, especially in the protein-rich tissues of hair, nails, muscle and skin. It assists in metabolism as a part of thiamine, biotin and pantothenic acid; helps regulate blood sugar levels as a constituent of insulin; and helps regulate blood clotting. Sulphur is also known to convert some toxic substances into non-toxic ones that can then be excreted, and therefore is used to treat poisoning from aluminum, cadmium, lead and mercury.

Any diet that provides sufficient protein is also providing adequate sulphur. Meat, fish, poultry, eggs, dairy products, peas and beans are rich in both nutrients. Neither sulphur deficiency nor toxicity occurs naturally in humans. Inorganic sulfur ingested in large amounts can be harmful, but excess organic sulphur from food is readily excreted. ■

Vanadium

RDA:
Not established

Vanadium is a trace mineral whose role in nutrition is uncertain but possibly essential. Evidence suggests that it lowers blood sugar levels in some people and inhibits tumour development, perhaps protecting against diabetes and some cancers. It also may contribute to cholesterol metabolism and hormone production. Vanadium exists in whole grains, nuts, root vegetables, liver, fish and vegetable oils. Because symptoms of its deficiency are unknown, it is assumed that humans need only a small amount, which diet apparently provides. ■

Zinc

RDA:
15 mg

The mineral zinc is integral to the synthesis of RNA and DNA, the genetic material that controls cell growth, division and function. In various proteins, enzymes, hormones and hormone-like substances called prostaglandins, zinc contributes to many bodily processes, including bone development and growth; cell respiration; energy metabolism; wound healing; the liver's ability to remove toxic substances such as alcohol from the body; immune function; and the regulation of heart rate and blood pressure. An adequate zinc intake enhances the ability to taste, promotes healthy skin and hair, enhances reproductive functions and may improve short-term memory and attention span. As an anti-inflammatory agent, zinc is sometimes used to treat acne, rheumatoid arthritis and prostatitis. Taking supplemental zinc may boost resistance to infection, especially in the elderly, and stimulate wound healing.

Zinc is most easily obtained from lean meat and seafood, but it is also found in eggs, soya beans, peanuts, wheat bran, cheese, oysters and other foods. Many Western diets are slightly low in zinc. Young children, pregnant women, vegetarians and elderly people are the most susceptible to zinc deficiency. Loss of taste is usually the first warning; other symptoms are hair loss or discoloration, white streaks on the nails, dermatitis, loss of appetite, fatigue and poor healing of wounds. In children, zinc deficiency can retard growth and stunt sexual development in boys. On the other hand, ingesting extreme amounts of zinc daily can impair immune function and cause nausea, headaches, vomiting, dehydration, stomach aches, poor muscle coordination, fatigue and possibly kidney failure. Experts recommend increasing zinc levels by increasing the zinc-rich foods in your diet or by taking a multi-nutrient supplement that includes zinc chelate, zinc picolinate or zinc aspartate, the three most easily absorbed forms. If zinc is used for more than three to six months to treat a chronic condition, it is essential to consult a nutritionist to avoid creating a mineral imbalance. Zinc ointment, which contains zinc oxide, is the most common topical form, and is useful for treating skin disorders, burns and other wounds. ■

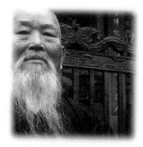

Target Ailments

- Back Problems
- Carpal Tunnel Syndrome
- Circulatory Problems
- Depression
- Hay Fever
- High Blood Pressure
- Insomnia
- Menopause Problems
- Neuralgia
- Pain, Chronic
- TMJ Syndrome

Qigong

Q igong ('chee-goong') is an ancient Chinese discipline that uses breathing exercises, movement and meditation to balance and strengthen the body's vital energy (chi, sometimes spelled 'qi'). Several of the martial arts, including t'ai chi (pages 139-140) and kung fu, are derived from qigong, but qigong itself is oriented more towards healing and less toward self-defence than these related practices.

Qigong, meaning 'energy cultivation', is intended to manipulate two forms of energy: internal chi and external chi. Internal chi can be developed by the repetition of qigong's ritual exercises and by meditation, a practice that is believed to balance the body's energies and promote internal well-being. Some qigong masters are said to be able to emit external chi, energy transmitted from one person to another for healing purposes.

Origins

Like many other forms of Chinese medicine, qigong dates back thousands of years. The modern practice of strengthening chi through ritual exercise and meditation contains strands of Buddhist, Taoist and Confucian philosophy developed over millennia. The Buddhist approach concentrates on freeing the self through awareness; the Taoist focuses on connection with the natural world; and the Confucian philosophy is more concerned with the place of the individual in society. Together they form the balance of inner and outer awareness that marks qigong today.

During China's Cultural Revolution in the 1960s and 1970s qigong was banned, but it later became clear that the discipline had millions of proponents in its native country. By the 1990s qigong was gaining popularity in the West as well.

What It's Good For

Qigong's supporters say that the practice can greatly improve overall health and even help cure a wide variety of ailments. In the years since the Cultural Revolution, China has hosted a number of medical conferences devoted to the healing effects of qigong. Papers presented at these meetings claim beneficial effects for ailments ranging from allergies and asthma to diabetes, hypertension, liver disorders and even paralysis and cancer. In more serious diseases, patients usually employ qigong along with conventional medical care to speed recovery and alleviate pain.

Preparations/Techniques

Those wishing to practise qigong should begin by studying with a teacher. The exercises are deceptively simple and need to be performed over and over again under

Qigong

the guidance of an expert before the student begins to feel their effects. There are literally thousands of qigong exercises, but the techniques can be divided into standing, sitting, lying and walking. Students may stand with legs apart and breathe from the diaphragm in a particular pattern while performing ritual movements with arms and legs; or they may sit and roll objects between their palms to stimulate energy points. Walking may be slow and regular, or more random and free. Students may also practise meditation techniques, focusing the mind on an energy point while counting breaths.

Between classes (which are taken once or twice a week), students go through the movements every day for about 30 minutes, morning and evening. Those who have particular medical problems may practise movements specific to their ailments for longer daily periods.

Some patients want to take the next step and visit a qigong master to experience the reputed healing power of external chi. These masters, more commonly found in China than in the West, believe that energy emitted from their hands passes into the patient's body, helping it to balance its own chi and heal its ailments. Such a master might touch or press specific 'chi points' on the body, or might pass his or her hands several inches above the body. Even these masters, however, will encourage patients to learn to develop internal chi so that they can take charge of their own health.

Well-being

Qigong, say its supporters, is a way of life. When practised every day, it is supposed to boost chi circulation and enhance overall health. Although people do turn to it for specific ailments, it is most properly used as a daily approach to well-being.

What the Critics Say

Because the medical research on qigong's health benefits is almost entirely Chinese, and critics claim that much of it does not conform to Western scientific standards, the Western medical establishment does not give much credence to qigong's reputed cures. The concept of external chi comes in for special criticism as being unlikely and unscientific. As with any form of medicine, conventional doctors urge the public to be extremely cautious of any practitioner making claims for 'miracle cures'. ■

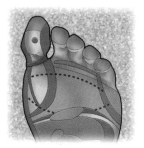

Target Ailments

- Anaemia
- Arthritis
- Back Problems
- Carpal Tunnel Syndrome
- Constipation
- Gout
- Hay Fever
- High Blood Pressure
- Ménière's Disease
- Motion Sickness
- Premenstrual Syndrome
- Stress
- Thyroid Problems

Reflexology

R eflexology involves the manipulation of specific areas on the feet—and sometimes on the hands or limbs—with the goal of bringing the body into homoeostasis, or balance. According to reflexologists, distinct regions of the feet correspond to particular organs or body systems. Stimulating the appropriate region with thumb or finger is intended to eliminate energy blockages thought to produce pain or disease in the associated structures. The arrangement of reflexology areas on the feet mirrors the organization of the body, to the extent that organs on the right side of the body are represented on the right foot, and so with the left.

Origins

The precise beginnings of reflexology are obscure, but the practice seems to have its roots in ancient Egypt as well as in Chinese medicine *(pages 45-48),* with its belief in energy pathways and body zones.

What It's Good For

The overall goal of reflexology is to balance the body's vital energies and thus promote overall health. Reflexologists maintain that their therapy helps improve blood supply, normalize overactive or underactive glands, unblock nerve impulses, and relieve stress. Although prevention, rather than cure, is the primary aim of reflexology, practitioners use it to relieve a wide variety of ailments, including headaches, sinus problems, constipation and insomnia.

Preparations/Techniques

Patients who want to try reflexology can visit a professional reflexologist for treatment. However, most people can also perform reflexology at home after studying the reflex areas and the techniques for working them.

Reflexologists divide the body into 10 longitudinal zones running from the head to the soles of the feet. By working a particular zone on the foot, proponents claim, you are affecting an organ within the corresponding zone in the upper body. The foot is further subdivided into specific reflex areas that relate to particular organs and structures, such as the eyes, liver and kidneys. Reflexologists recognize nearly 30 areas on the sole of each foot *(see the illustration on page 138).*

Reflexology features techniques that can be performed either by yourself or by a partner. The basic thumb technique uses the inside edge of the thumb pad (the side away from the fingers) to 'walk' along reflex areas; walking consists of a forward, creeping movement, with the first joint of the thumb bending and unbending slightly as the digit inches ahead. The finger technique uses the same walking mo-

Reflexology

tion but with the edge of the index finger next to the thumb. When working an area, one hand should work and the other should hold the foot in a comfortable position with the sole flat and the toes straight. As they work each reflex area, reflexologists feel for tension or minute grainy spots, or 'crystals', beneath the skin, believing that these are signs of blockages or pain in the relevant part of the body. The thumb and finger techniques aim to remove the tension and these crystals.

Some reflexologists also teach that the hands and other so-called referral areas can be worked in the same way. In hand reflexology, the thumb of one hand works the palm of the other; the index finger works the areas between the fingers and the V between the thumb and the index finger of the opposite hand. Referral areas are places on the body thought to have an anatomical similarity to the afflicted area. For instance, the elbow would be the referral area for the knee, the wrist for the ankle. If a patient sprained a right ankle, a reflexologist might work the right wrist in addition to, or in place of, the corresponding area on the foot.

Well-being

Reflexologists view their therapy as preventive maintenance. Daily practice of its techniques, they say, can keep the body running smoothly. Like the ancient physicians who went before them, reflexologists believe that a person who pursues well-being by balancing the body's energies and relaxing stress and tension will rarely fall sick.

What the Critics Say

Many conventional medical practitioners dismiss reflexology as an example of 'magical thinking'—the belief that objects can be influenced simply by thinking about them. Sceptics also point out that reflexologists have not established any sci-entific basis for asserting that the feet or hands are connected in a therapeutic way with other parts of the body. To some critics, in fact, reflexology treatments are noth-ing more than glorified foot massages. Proponents, however, maintain that the health benefits of reflexology are extensive and well documented. ∎

FOR MORE INFO
Following are twoorganizations you can contact to learn more about reflexology:

Association of Reflexologists
27 Old Gloucester Street
London WC1N 3XX
0870 567 3320
website: www.reflexology.org/aor

Bailey School of **Reflexology**
Monks Orchard
Whitbourne
Worcester WR6 5RB
01886 821 207
Fax: 01886 822 017

CONTINUED

REFLEXOLOGY AREAS

Right and Left Bottom
1. Brain
2. Sinus, Head, Brain
3. Side, Neck
4. Pituitary, Pineal
5. Eyes, Ears
6. Throat, Neck, Thyroid
7. Oesophagus
8. Thymus
9. Heart
10. Lung, Breast
11. Arm
12. Thyroid, Bronchi
13. Shoulder
14. Solar Plexus
15. Diaphragm
16. Adrenal Glands
17. Gall bladder
18. Liver
19. Stomach
20. Duodenum
21. Kidneys
22. Waistline
23. Pancreas
24. Transverse Colon
25. Ureters
26. Ascending Colon
27. Bladder
28. Small Intestine
29. Sacrum, Coccyx
30. Sciatic
31. Sigmoid Colon
32. Ileocoecal Valve, Appendix
33. Descending Colon
34. Spleen

Right Outside, Left Inside
35. Sciatic
36. Pelvic Area
37. Hip, Back, Sciatic
38. Ovary, Testicle
39. Prostate, Uterus, Rectum, Sciatic
40. Lymph, Groin, Fallopian Tube
41. Uterus, Prostate
42. Bladder
43. Breast, Lung
44. Sinus, Head, Brain
45. Arm, Shoulder
46. Lower Back
47. Sacrum, Coccyx
48. Lumbar
49. Thoracic
50. Cervical

Right and Left Top
51. Lymph, Groin, Fallopian Tube
52. Knee, Leg, Hip, Lower Back
53. Chest, Lung, Breast, Back
54. Chest, Lung, Breast, Back, Heart

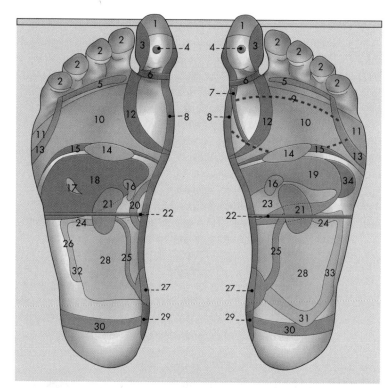

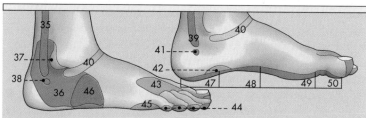

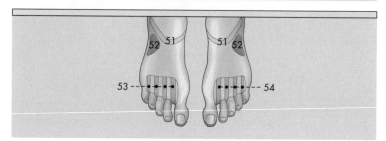

T'ai Chi

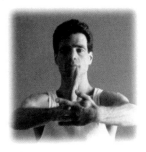

T'ai chi ch'uan—commonly known as t'ai chi—is an ancient Chinese practice that combines martial arts, exercise, and meditation in one graceful, slow-motion art. Every morning in parks across Asia, and increasingly in the West as well, practitioners of t'ai chi perform what appears to be a trance-like, controlled dance. This dance is in fact a combination of t'ai chi 'forms'—ritual movements intended to promote the flow of internal energy, increase self-awareness, and strengthen and relax the body.

Though often considered more a martial art than a therapeutic technique, t'ai chi provides many health benefits, including improved strength, flexibility and relaxation. The ritual movements are meant to move the body's energy (chi—sometimes spelled 'qi') to its natural centre, called the tan t'ien, about 2 in (5 cm) below the navel. The energy is then said to circulate throughout the body, correcting existing conditions and preventing illness.

Target Ailments

- Arthritis
- Back Problems
- Bronchitis
- Cholesterol Problems
- Depression
- Hay Fever
- Headache
- Insomnia
- Neuralgia
- Osteoporosis
- Pain, Chronic
- Stress
- Tendinitis
- Wind and Painful Wind

Origins

T'ai chi's roots reach down thousands of years to the origins of Eastern philosophy itself. Many of its principles are found in the *Tao Tê Ching,* traditionally written by the sage Lao-tzu (604-531 BC). Taoist philosophy holds that *tao*—'the way'— is the force that gives shape and energy to all things, and that to understand tao one must understand one's place in the natural world. Chinese doctors and martial artists alike incorporated Taoist and then Buddhist views into their practices, developing ritual exercises that mimicked the natural movements of animals such as the horse, the tiger and the crane.

By the 19th century, the modern forms of t'ai chi were brought to Beijing, where they quickly became popular. Chinese immigrants then took the art to the West. In recent years t'ai chi has gained a considerable following outside China.

What It's Good For

Advocates of t'ai chi discourage its use as a remedy for specific ills. Instead, they say, the art is intended to correct imbalances in one's life and to strengthen inner energy, so that those who practise it feel calm, harmonious and invigorated. The positive effects of this slow, intense exercise include improved muscle strength, particularly in the lower body, better flexibility, better posture and balance, and relaxation. Proponents say the exercise may also prevent sleeplessness, backache and the pain of arthritis. Because it is slow and can be practised so as not to stress joints, t'ai chi is good exercise for children and the elderly.

CONTINUED

T'ai Chi CONTINUED

Preparations/Techniques

Newcomers to t'ai chi are advised to study the art with an experienced teacher. Classes can be found through local YMCAs, health clubs, Taoist centres and in the Yellow Pages under 'Martial Arts'. A class might begin with meditation and warm-ups, proceed to work on specific forms and end with a cool-down. The slow, lissome movements look deceptively easy; in fact, they require serious concentration and control, and participants will work up a sweat. Progress takes time. Although some of the forms can be learned in a few weeks, students typically need one or two years to achieve the state of relaxed alertness and control of detail that t'ai chi requires.

Students should attend class at least once a week and then practise at home every day. The movements require only a modest amount of flat, open space. Many people like to practise in the morning, when they are alert and fresh, or in the evening, as a way to unwind after a stressful day. Experts recommend exercising in the open air, if possible; the fresh air and tranquillity are conducive to a peaceful state of mind, and some advocates feel that energy travels more freely in a natural setting.

T'ai chi forms are combinations of stances that flow continuously into one another. 'Short forms' might have as few as 24 postures; a 'long form' would have up to 88.

Well-being

T'ai chi, like other Chinese arts, is devoted to well-being. Incorporating physical, mental and spiritual exercise, t'ai chi's mission is to invigorate both body and mind and clear the flow of energy. In that way, proponents claim, t'ai chi practitioners can live into old age strong and free of disease.

What the Critics Say

The concept of chi—energy flowing through channels in the body—is not accepted by everyone. Critics note that there is no scientific evidence for such an energy flow. But even critics acknowledge that t'ai chi exercises are unlikely to do harm—and, like any exercise, quite probably do some good. ∎

FOR MORE INFO

Following is an organization you can contact to learn more about t'ai chi:

Tai Chi Union for Great Britain
69 Kilpatrick Gardens
Clarkston
Glasgow G76 7RF
0141 638 2946
fax: 0141 621 1220
email: taichi@dial.pipex.com
website:
http://dspace.dial.pipex.com/taichi

Taichi Qigong Health Centre
01493 601111
email: colinorr@taichi-qigong.net

Yoga

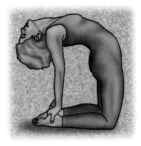

Yoga is an ancient philosophy of life developed in India over the course of thousands of years. The word 'yoga' is derived from the Sanskrit 'yuj', which means union. Practitioners of yoga believe that by following its precepts, which include ethical principles, dietary restrictions, and physical exercise, they can unite—or bring into equilibrium—the mind, the body and the spirit. According to yoga teaching, physical illness is a sign that these elements are out of balance.

There are many different forms of yoga. Hatha-yoga, widely practised in the West, consists of a series of body positions and movements, known as asanas, and breathing exercises, called pranayama. Many Western practitioners also include relaxation and meditation in their daily yoga routine.

Origins

No one knows exactly when people in India began practising yoga, but small stone carvings of figures in yogic postures, thought to be more than 5,000 years old, have been excavated in the Indus Valley. In the third century BC, the sage Patanjali wrote the Yoga Sutras, verses that describe eight steps to spiritual enlightenment. The postures and breathing techniques in the Yoga Sutras form the foundation of the modern practice of hatha-yoga.

What It's Good For

Yoga is thought to be a powerful health enhancer, helping the body become stronger and more resilient against disease and injuries. The postures stretch and strengthen muscles, massage internal organs, relax nerves and increase blood circulation. Because yoga can work every muscle, nerve, and gland in the body, it is used to treat and prevent a wide array of conditions and illnesses.

- **Athletic injuries:** Athletes from long-distance runners to professional football players use yoga stretches to keep the body agile and the muscles injury free.
- **Back problems:** Because yoga postures flex, tone and strengthen muscles, they are often prescribed for chronic back problems.
- **Heart problems:** Studies have shown that performing yoga can help the heart work more efficiently. It can also aid in lowering blood pressure and cholesterol levels.
- **Stress:** Regular yoga practice has been found to reduce feelings of anxiety, anger, fatigue and depression.

Target Ailments

- Asthma
- Athletic Injuries
- Back Problems
- Cancer
- Chronic Fatigue Syndrome
- Depression
- Diabetes
- Glandular Fever
- Headache
- Heart Problems
- High Blood Pressure
- Indigestion
- Irritable Bowel Syndrome
- Menstrual Problems
- Pain, Chronic
- Premenstrual Syndrome
- Sore Throat
- Stress

CONTINUED

Yoga CONTINUED

CAUTION

Some of the more advanced, upside-down yoga postures, such as headstands, can be dangerous for people with high blood pressure or eye problems. Pregnant women should avoid postures that compress or strain the abdomen or back.

FOR MORE INFO
Followingare organizations you can contact to learn more about yoga:

British Wheel of Yoga
1 Hamilton Place
Boston Road
Sleaford
Lincolnshire NG34 7ES
01529 306 851
fax: 01529 303 233

Yoga for Health Foundation
Ickwell Bury
Biggleswade
Bedfordshire SG18 9EF
01767 627 271
fax: 01767 627 266

The Kevala Centre
Hunsdon Road
Torquay
Devon TQ1 1QB
01803 215 678
email: information@kevala.co.uk
website: www.kevala.co.uk

Preparations/Techniques

Yoga can be performed with an instructor or alone. Experts recommend that you set aside at least half an hour each day, preferably in the morning or late evening, primarily because the postures should be done on an empty stomach. Choose a clean, warm area with a level floor. Wear loose clothing.

Begin with a few minutes of deep breathing to draw energy and oxygen into your body and help calm your mind. Follow with a few warm-up exercises, then practise the postures you have chosen for that day's session. Go slowly and gently; no posture should cause extreme or increased pain. End each session with five to 10 minutes of relaxation.

Visiting a Professional

To find an instructor, check the phone book to see if your community has a yoga centre. Yoga classes are also offered in many health clubs, hospitals, and community centres. When choosing a yoga teacher for class or individual instruction, find one who practices yoga daily and who studies regularly with a teacher of his or her own. Your teacher should also be knowledgeable about major muscle groups and body systems and should tailor yoga techniques to your individual capability.

Well-being

Daily yoga practice offers a gentle and effective way of achieving good health and staying well. Practitioners believe that because yoga calms the mind as well as the body, it can prevent many chronic stress-related diseases and conditions.

What the Critics Say

Although acknowledging yoga's many beneficial effects, critics worry that people will injure themselves by jumping into yoga too enthusiastically and attempting advanced postures for which they have not adequately prepared their body. They are also concerned that people will use yoga instead of, rather than as a complement to, conventional medicine for serious conditions such as cancer and diabetes. Most yoga experts share these concerns and stress that beginners should start with easy postures and gradually work toward more difficult ones. They also advise people with pre-existing conditions to check with their doctor before trying any postures. ■

Index

Page numbers in italic refer to illustrations or to illustrated text.